"The scope is impressive. The editors have acknowledged and addressed the range of issues that a hospice confronts when beginning to provide care for persons with AIDS. The issues have been grounded in reality through the implementation of studies to systematically examine each issue. This is an interesting approach that goes beyond the more common case study description of care needs. This book will be useful manual on the shelf not only of hospice agencies, but also of individual hospice professionals."

—Helen Schietinger, RN, Consultant to domestic and international agencies in HIV policy, care, and prevention

AIDS
and the Hospice Community

AIDS
and the Hospice
Community

Madalon O'Rawe Amenta
Editor

with the assistance of
Claire B. Tehan

AIDS and the Hospice Community was simultaneously issued by The Haworth Press, Inc., under the same title, as a special issue of *The Hospice Journal,* Volume 7, Numbers 1/2 1991, Madalon O'Rawe Amenta, Editor, with the assistance of Claire B. Tehan.

Harrington Park Press
An Imprint of The Haworth Press, Inc.
New York • London • Sydney

ISBN 1-56023-011-8

Published by

Harrington Park Press, 10 Alice Street, Binghamton, NY 13904-1580
EUROSPAN/Harrington, 3 Henrietta Street, London WC2E 8LU England
ASTAM/Harrington, 162-168 Parramatta Road, Stanmore, Sydney, N.S.W. 2048 Australia

Harrington Park Press is an imprint of The Haworth Press, Inc., 10 Alice Street, Binghamton, NY 13904-1580.

AIDS and the Hospice Community was originally published as *The Hospice Journal*, Volume 7, Numbers 1/2 1991.

Library of Congress Cataloging-in-Publication Data

AIDS and the hospice community / Madalon O'Rawe Amenta, editor.
    p. cm.
    "Simultaneously issued by The Haworth Press, Inc. under the same title as a special issue of The Hospice Journal, volume 7, numbers 1/2, 1991.
    ISBN 1-56023-011-8 (HPP : alk. paper).
    1. AIDS (Disease)—Palliative treatment. 2. Hospice care. I. Amenta, Madalon O'Rawe.
    [DNLM: 1. Acquired Immunodeficiency Syndrome. 2. Hospices. WD 308 A28785]
RC607.A26A34564   1991b
362.1'9697'92—dc20
DNLM/DLC
for Library of Congress   91-20899
                                              CIP

CONTENTS

ABOUT THE EDITORS

Madalon O'Rawe Amenta, RN, DPH, Associate Professor of Nursing at The Pennsylvania State University, McKeesport Campus, has long been active in the hospice field as an organizer, educator, researcher, writer, and editor. She is Vice-President of the Hospice Nurses Association and Chairperson of the Professional Advisory Committee of Home Health Services of Allegheny County. Previously, she was Director of Research and Education at the Forbes Hospice in Pittsburgh, founded and served as the first President of the Pennsylvania Hospice Network, and was Mid-Atlantic Region Representative to the Board of Directors of the National Hospice Organization. The author of over fifty articles, chapters, and sets of standards, and editor of several professional and organizational newsletters, Dr. Amenta is the co-author, with Nancy Bohnet, of the prize-winning book *Nursing Care of the Terminally Ill.*

Claire Tehan, MA, has been Vice President for Hospice at Hospital Home Health Care Agency of California since 1977. She is also Chair of the National Hospice Organization AIDS Resource Committee and President of the California State Hospice Association. Active in the American hospice movement since 1975, she has served six years on the National Hospice Organization Board of Directors.

AIDS
and the Hospice Community

Preface

Even though statistics compiled by the National Hospice Organization in its annual surveys indicate substantial and growing numbers of AIDS patients being served in hospices throughout the nation, there is still a perception that the relationship of the hospice community and the AIDS epidemic has been, and remains a tentative, if not an uneasy one. There seem to be natural barriers to cooperation inherent in both the organizational characteristics of contemporary hospices as well as in the nature of the AIDS disease progression and the attitudes of persons with AIDS toward treatment and the goals of treatment.

At what point can AIDS patients be certified to be in a terminal stage? How are curative and/or palliative therapies defined? Do AIDS patients fit a hospice's eligibility criteria? Can they be incorporated into its mission? Is the average hospice, usually a small organization, capable of accommodating the intense acuity of care — physical as well as psychosocial — of AIDS patients? Will a hospice put itself in financial jeopardy by assuming an AIDS caseload? How will staff and volunteers be affected by the fear of infection? How will the widespread social stigma associated with AIDS affect volunteer recruitment and retention? How will it affect customary fund raising resources in the community?

Despite these ambiguities, many members of the hospice community have been exploring and experimenting. In this volume there are descriptions and findings from research projects carried out in urban and rural hospice programs, and one in a federal prison, that document the social stigma, staff and volunteer stress, and lack of social support that can accompany the care of terminally ill AIDS patients. There are findings about the attitudes of rural nurses that indicate a need for attitudinal education as well as for technical information about AIDS and hospice care. This study also points up the need for educational and resource preparation of rural physicians and health care facilities before the heaviest impact of the spread of the AIDS epidemic from the urban coastal centers to the heartland is realized. There is an account of a model program for dealing with infection control and confidentiality policies and practices in the workplace. There is a description of some of the special bereavement concerns of persons with AIDS and their families and friends. There is also a compendium of tested print and audio-visual resources about AIDS for various hospice program uses from policy formation, to education of staff and volunteers, to education of the community. Finally, there are examples of hospice programs that in extending themselves to caring for AIDS patients and participating in AIDS support groups have moved awareness of the hospice philosophy further in their communities than ever before.

We do not in this volume resolve any issues. We formalize the acknowledgment of them. We specify indicators of willingness to embrace the challenge on the part of various local hospices, professionals, and volunteers, and we present examples of agencies that are actively giving care to persons with AIDS and their families and friends. We also acknowledge the concern at the national level expressed in the work of the National Hospice Organization's AIDS Resource Committee, chaired by Claire Tehan. She was instrumental in the conception of this volume and in the solicitation of several of its articles from members of the committee.

In sum, we document the facts. In the midst of profound questions and uncertainties the hospice spirit is reaching out. The hospice community is doing with AIDS what it did originally, only a little more than a decade ago, with death and dying — translating its vision into the daily workings of the possible. That is the provision of hands on care in grass roots communities all across the country. There are many forms this concerned action takes and many conceivable organizational structures will result. In the meantime, the hospice community keeps working at it.

Madalon O'Rawe Amenta

Some Notes on the Impact
of Treating AIDS Patients
in Hospices

Robert J. Miller

SUMMARY. As part of a larger nation-wide study of attitudes of hospice personnel, we incorporated questions about patient autonomy and economic justice in which we asked the respondents to share their beliefs about AIDS patients compared to patients terminally ill with other diagnoses. The convenience sample of 826 hospice workers, 76% of whom were clinical professionals (nurses, physicians, social workers) rated terminally ill patients and those with AIDS the same in terms of right to refuse life sustaining medical therapy. Although over one half believed that we are not currently spending enough on the care of AIDS patients, 25% thought that we spend too much on those terminally ill with other diagnoses. Issues of survival time, costs of care, and staff concerns about treating AIDS patients in hospices are briefly discussed.

INTRODUCTION

At the time the first large groups of AIDS patients were becoming terminally ill in the 1980s, American hospice programs were treating a fairly homogeneous population of elderly, middle class, white patients dying of cancer. There was some doubt if AIDS patients belonged in hospice. Nonetheless, some hospice programs

---

Robert J. Miller, MD, is Medical Director of the St. Anthony's Cancer Care Center in St. Petersburg, FL; Chairman of the Physician's Advisory Committee for Hospice Care, Inc. of Pinellas County, FL; and was the first President of the Academy of Hospice Physicians.

Address correspondence to the author at Bayfront Cancer Care Center, 701 6th St. South, St. Petersburg, FL 33701.

took the lead in reaching out and caring for these people, and hospices now care for a sizable and ever increasing number.

According to the National Hospice Organization, (I. Bates, personal communication, January 3, 1991) in 1989, hospices provided some care for 8,048 people with AIDS or 33% of all U.S. AIDS deaths in that year. This number represented 4.3% of the 186,719 patients served in 1989 by American hospices. As of May 1990 there were 136,204 cases of AIDS/HIV disease and 83,145 deaths (Pickett, Drewry, & Comer, 1990) and an estimated one to two million infected Americans (Bartlett, 1990). As the numbers mount, the pressures on hospices will increase. Hospice directors will have to face the modifications they may need to make in their programs if they are to meet the intense clinical, psychosocial, and economic demands characteristic of these, heretofore, "nontraditional" hospice patients and their families.

How are persons with AIDS viewed in comparison with patients terminally ill with cancer within the hospice community? And what are the perceived and real financial consequences of treating these patients? In order to find out about these issues we incorporated questions about them into a larger survey of attitudes of hospice personnel we conducted in 1990.

THE SURVEY

The Questionnaire

We developed the survey questions and field tested them with local hospice staff and then ascertained content validity by having three national expert consultants review them. We mailed the questionnaire to all 600 active members of the Academy of Hospice Physicians in March, 1990. The staffs of three hospices, two in Florida and one in Texas, two of which serve combined urban and rural populations and one that is largely urban, were also asked to complete it. And lastly, we distributed it with the 1990 Spring issue of the *American Journal of Hospice and Palliative Care*, a national publication subscribed to by many in the hospice community.

The Sample

The number of completed surveys returned from the three sources from which this convenience sample was compiled was 826. Four hundred eighty-eight (59%) came from the readers of the journal, 209 (25%) from the members of the Academy of Hospice Physicians, and 111 (13%) from the 3 hospices in Florida and Texas.

Forty-one percent of the respondents were nurses, 29% physicians, 12% administrators, 6% social workers, 4% volunteers, and 6% others. It is noteworthy that 76% of this sample — nurses, physicians, social workers — were clinical professionals.

Patient Autonomy

In the matter of patient autonomy, it can be inferred from study of Table 1 that when hospice workers think of a competent patient's right to refuse life sustaining medical therapy, those with AIDS are viewed in the same way as are patients with terminal cancer. Ninety-nine percent of the respondents thought each group should have the right to refuse, despite the younger age of terminally ill AIDS patients, uncertainties about their prognosis, and higher probability that their disease may involve neurological and brain lesions. The respondents saw it somewhat differently, however, (82% agreeing) when it came to autonomous decision making for competent patients with conditions such as Alzheimer's Disease, and substantially differently (24% agreeing) for depressed patients.

Economic Justice

In the area of economic justice or the fair and equitable distribution of health care resources, several points stood out. In general these respondents from the hospice community (86%) agreed that "the health care team has a responsibility to serve the best interest of the patient, even in a world of limited resources." Only 5% clearly disagreed and 9% were not sure. When it came to very expensive treatments for terminally ill patients that "might" have "some benefit" for the patient, however, only 14% of these hospice worker respondents thought that only the patient should be

Table 1 Beliefs of Hospice Workers About Rights of Competent Patients to Refuse Life Sustaining Medical Therapy

PATIENT'S CONDITION	Has Right		Does Not Have Right		Not Sure		Total
	N	%*	N	%*	N	%*	N
Terminal cancer	810	99	2	0.25	3	0.37	815
AIDS	810	99	4	0.50	2	0.25	816
Quadraplegic	720	89	34	4.00	58	7.00	812
Early Alzheimer's	662	82	50	6.00	100	12.00	812
For Religious Reasons (e.g. Jehovah's Witness)	533	66	117	15.00	151	19.00	801
Pregnant	356	44	201	25.00	255	31.00	812
Severely depressed	194	24	340	42.00	276	34.00	810

* Percentages are based on totals of those responding to each item

considered. Thirty-four percent thought the patient and the family should be considered in the decision and the largest percentage (44%) advocated considering the patient, the family, and society.

As to the amount of money presently being spent on AIDS care, there did not seem to be evidence of bias against AIDS patients. Quite the opposite (see Table 2). Whereas 27% of the respondents thought we were already spending too much on terminally ill patients, only 5% believed we were spending too much money on those with AIDS. It is important to note that about one-third of the respondents were unsure about each of these issues.

DISCUSSION

It would appear from the answers to these questions, that a large number of hospice clinical professionals in this country think that patients with AIDS should have a high degree of autonomy in making medical decisions about their own care. If amount being spent is an indicator, these respondents think AIDS patients are not receiving enough care resources. Might one infer compassion and a call to action?

How is the hospice organizational/managerial community responding? At present, there would seem to be a distinct 'approach/avoidance' attitude about the matter. Persons with AIDS do not fit the accustomed pattern of 'traditional hospice patients' with predictable, limited survival time, and a willingness to forgo intensive life prolonging therapy and accept only palliative, supportive care. Persons with AIDS also raise other potentially troublesome issues.

Survival Time

Prior to the advent of current therapy the median survival time for persons diagnosed with AIDS was 28 weeks (Bartlett, 1990). Survival after the first episode of pneumocystis pneumonia has been improving and now approaches 2 years (Redfield & Tramont, 1989; Harris, 1990; Lemp, Payne, Rutherford et al., 1990; Fischl, Richman, Causey et al., 1989). A recent series of patients treated with AZT (zidovudine) had a median survival of 21.3 months (Lemp, Payne, Neal et al., 1990). It is likely with the application of increas-

Table 2
Beliefs About Amounts of Money Currently Expended on
Terminally Ill and AIDS Patients

TYPE OF PATIENT	Too Much		About Right		Not Enough		Unsure		Total
	N	%*	N	%*	N	%*	N	%*	N
Terminally Ill	220	27	111	14	234	29	242	30	807
AIDS	45	5	80	10	434	54	249	31	808

* Percentages are based on totals of those responding to each item.

6

ing clinical expertise resulting from ongoing research that survival time will continue to improve (Bennett, Garfinkle, Greenfield et al., 1989). Much more information is needed before we can begin to predict approximate six month survival (Justice, Feinstein, & Wells, 1989; Ragni & Kingsley, 1989). What can be said at present is that physicians have difficulty in certifying AIDS patients as having a prognosis of six months or less, therefore these patients may often be excluded from programs such as Medicare and Medicaid that have such requirements.

Even though many of these patients live longer than six months, it is clear from the results of this survey that the hospice clinical professional community considers them terminally ill. Other studies have demonstrated that a variety of health care workers, not just those in hospices, view persons with AIDS this way as well (Wachter, Luce, Hearst, & Lo, 1989). Even if these patients live longer than six months and many still desire what might appear to traditional hospice workers to be intensive therapy for increasing their survival time, there is no denying their desperate need for the type of psychosocial and supportive care that hospice provides. What is needed is a better definition of what constitutes the hospice philosophy and a more realistic interpretation of palliative care. At present, most of the "intensive" treatments that AIDS patients seek, are truly palliative.

Economic Issues

The economic impact of the AIDS epidemic is expected to be great with hospitals losing considerable money on both inpatient and outpatient care (Andrulis, Weslowski & Gage, 1989; Fineberg 1988). With the increasing life expectancy of patients all through the disease spectrum, from diagnosis of HIV infection through actual AIDS to death, based on estimated total cost of $85,333 per case, total medical costs are likely to rise from $4.1-5.4 billion in 1990 to $6.5-11 billion by 1994 (American Medical News, July 20, 1990; p.3).

With better use of community resources it may be possible to keep costs down. The average medical costs for the first 10,000 AIDS patients in the United States in 1986 was $147,000 (Hardy,

Rauch, Echenberg et al., 1986). But an analysis of the costs of patients treated at San Francisco General Hospital during 1984, with its strong community support system revealed an average cost of only $27,571 (Scitovsky, Cline, & Lee, 1986). In 1987 the average lifetime costs were estimated to be $65,000-$80,000 (Pickett, Drewry, & Comer, 1990), and current estimates are $40,000-$75,000 (Green & Arno, 1990). Estimates of total costs are apt to vary widely as the treatment and outcome of this disease change rapidly. Estimates also vary at present because of the differences in resources available from community to community and state to state.

The Florida Experience

For purposes of illustrating potential AIDS patient volume we will take the experience of treating AIDS in community hospices in Sarasota, Tampa, and Orlando—all in West Central Florida—as representative of what may be expected across the country. The accumulated incidence of AIDS cases in these counties is slightly higher than the national average. In all three programs there has been an increasing number of AIDS hospice patients that reflects the rising prevalence of AIDS in the community. In a relatively low incidence area such as Sarasota with a total accumulated incidence of AIDS of 73.9/100,000 as of 11/30/90, persons with AIDS diagnoses make up approximately 2%-4% of all hospice patients. In Orlando with a total accumulated incidence of 112/100,000, they constitute 4-8% of all hospice patients. In Tampa, a more urban area, where the incidence is higher (113/100,000) 11% of hospice patients have AIDS.

It is generally acknowledged that the cost of treating AIDS patients in hospices can amount to twice the cost of treating patients with other diagnoses, especially when medication costs are taken into consideration. But there is documentation of a growing tendency for AIDS patients to rely on Medicaid for funding (Green & Arno, 1990). In Florida, starting in 1990, a Medicaid Waiver program was implemented through the state health department. Under its terms, AIDS patients who are not considered to have six months or less to live may receive hospice care without losing their basic

Medicaid coverage which includes payment for medication. Some hospices have begun using this program and others are searching for other sources of funding to pay for medication costs.

The Clinical Challenge

That AIDS patients and their families require more intensive levels of support services and that the patients, themselves, are more difficult to treat clinically than are traditional hospice patients is well known. These patients are relatively young. Many present pain control difficulty because of a long-standing history of drug abuse. More than half of them have severe and persistent diarrheas. Others have progressive dementia and blindness. Additionally there are the psychosocial problems of life style issues, and lack of traditional, and in some cases "alternative" family support (Librach, 1987). Some of these patients are totally abandoned. They suffer social stigmatization, and because of life style issues have an increased need for confidentiality and privacy (Gilmore, 1987).

Hospice Staff Issues

While the patients cope with the physical realities of the disease and the stigma and fear which society imposes on them, the hospice staff needs to deal with the guilt, shame, or anger they may feel in identification with the patients (Carr, 1989). There are also many demanding ethical issues for staff: managing truth, confidentiality, cessation of treatment, refusal of treatment, suicide and euthanasia that are much more common with these patients (Morissette, 1990; Kizer, Green, Perkins et al., 1988).

The risk of contagion. The risk of contagion to the health care staff is an issue critical to the acceptance of persons with AIDS within traditional hospices. Whereas the risk of infection has been considered low, (Ciesielski, Bell, Chamberland et al., 1990; Decker & Schaffner, 1986; Lifson, Castro, McCray, & Jaffee, 1986) we have to acknowledge that it is real (Gerberding, Littell, Tarkington et al., 1990; Kelen, DiBiovanna, Bisson et al., 1989). The impact—devastating psychologically, socially, physically, financially—when a health care worker becomes exposed or infected has been graphically described (Aoun, 1989; Henry, Jackson, Balfour et al., 1990).

Because of these obvious and other more subtle reasons many health care workers remain extremely uncomfortable about the prospect of caring for people with AIDS (Cooke & Sande, 1989; Gerbert, Maguire, Badner et al., 1988). There is, then, an urgent need to both support and protect the rights of the health care staff (Dickey, 1989; Rhame, 1990; Volberding, 1989).

CONCLUSION

The AIDS epidemic is forcing many hospice programs to reexamine their philosophy of care and redefine the role of hospice in caring for the dying. Caring for AIDS patients is a challenge that requires learning new clinical skills, dealing with different types of stress, and negotiating the financial resources necessary to provide optimal care. The experience to date suggests that the hospice system of care is an appropriate one for caring for AIDS patients, that the hospice spirit—as exemplified in the respondents to this survey—is willing, and that many hospices are already striving to concretely define and to actively meet the challenge.

REFERENCES

Andrulis, D.P., Weslowski, V.B., & Gage, L.S. (1989). The 1987 U.S. hospital AIDS survey. *Journal of the American Medical Association, 262*, 784-794.

Aoun, H. (1989). When a house officer get AIDS. *New England Journal of Medicine, 321*, 693-696.

Bartlett, J. (1990). Current and future treatment of HIV infection. *Oncology, 4* (11), 19-29.

Bennett, C.L., Garfinkle, J.B., Greenfield, S. et al. (1989). The relation between hospital experience and in-hospital mortality for patients with AIDS-related PCP. *Journal of the American Medical Association, 261*, 2975-2979.

Carr, E.W. (1989). Psychosocial issues of AIDS patients in hospice: case studies. *The Hospice Journal, 5* (3/4), 135-151.

Ciesielski, C.A., Bell, D.M., Chamberland, M.E. et al. (letter). (1990). *New England Journal of Medicine, 322*, 1156.

Cooke, M., & Sande, M.A. (1989). The HIV epidemic and training in internal medicine. Challenges and recommendations. *New England Journal of Medicine, 321*, 1334-8.

Decker, M., & Schaffner, W. (1986). Risk of AIDS to health care workers. *Journal of the American Medical Association, 256*, 3264-3265.

Dickey, N.W. (1989). Physicians and acquired immunodeficiency syndrome: a reply to patients. *Journal of the American Medical Association, 262*, 2002-2003.

Fineberg, H.V. (1988). The social dimensions of AIDS. *Scientific American*, October, pp. 128-134.

Fischl, M.A., Richman, D.D., Causey, D.M. et al. (1989). Prolonged Zidovudine therapy in patients with AIDS and advanced AIDS-related complex. *Journal of the American Medical Association, 262*, 2405-2410.

Gerberding, J.F., Littell, C., Tarkington, A. et al. (1990). Risk of exposure of surgical personnel to patients' blood during surgery at San Francisco General Hospital. *New England Journal of Medicine, 322*, 1788-1793.

Gerbert, B., Maguire, B., Badner, V. et al. (1988). Why fear persists: health care professionals and AIDS. *Journal of the American Medical Association, 260*, 3481-3483.

Gilmore, N. (1987). AIDS palliative care: the courage to care. *Journal of Palliative Care, 3* (2), 33-38.

Hardy, A.M., Rauch, K., Echenberg, D. et al. (1986). The economic impact of the first 10,000 cases of acquired immunodeficiency syndrome in the United States. *Journal of the American Medical Association, 255*, 209-211.

Harris, J.E. (1990). Improved short-term survival of AIDS patients initially diagnosed with Pneumocystic carinii pneumonia, 1984 through 1987. *Journal of the American Medical Association, 263*, 397-401.

Henderson, D.K., Beekmann, S.E., & Gerberding, J. (1990). Post-exposure antiviral chemoprophylaxis following occupational exposure to the Human Immunodeficiency virus. *AIDS Updates, 3*, 1-8.

Henry, K., Jackson, B., Balfour, H. et al. (1990). Long-term follow-up of health care workers with work-site exposure to human immunodeficiency virus. (letter) *New England Journal of Medicine, 322*, 1765-6.

Justice, A.C., Feinstein, A.R., & Wells, C.K. (1989). A new prognostic staging system for the acquired immunodeficiency syndrome. *New England Journal of Medicine, 320*, 1388-1393.

Kelen, G.D., DiGiovanna, T., Bisson, T. et al. (1989). Human immunodeficiency virus infection in emergency department patients. Epidemiology, clinical presentations, and risk to health care workers: The Johns Hopkins experience. *Journal of the American Medical Association, 262*, 516-522.

Kizer, K., Green, M., Perkins, C. et al. (1988). AIDS and suicide in California. *Journal of the American Medical Association, 260*, 1881.

Lemp, G.F., Payne, S.F., Rutherford, G.W. et al. (1990). Projections of AIDS morbidity and mortality in San Francisco. *Journal of the American Medical Association, 263*, 1497-1501.

Lemp, G.F., Payne, S.F., Neal, D. et al. (1990). Survival trends for patients with AIDS. *Journal of the American Medical Association, 263*, 402-406.

Librach, S.L. (1987). Acquired immunodeficiency syndrome: the challenge for palliative care. *Journal of Palliative Care, 3* (2), 31-33.

Lifson, A., Castro, K., McCray, E., & Jaffe, H., (1986). National surveillance of AIDS in health care workers. *Journal of the American Medical Association, 256,* 3231-3234.

Morissette, M.R. (1990). AIDS and palliative care: an individual appeal to health care professionals and intervening parties. *Journal of Palliative Care, 6* (1), 26-31.

Pickett, N.A., Dewry, S.J., & Comer, E.L. (1990). Metropolitan life insurance company's experience with AIDS, in *Statistical Bulletin,* October-December 1990, as reported in Oncology, *4* (11), 32-38.

Ragni, M.V., Kingsley, L.A. (1989). Importance of age in prognostic staging system for AIDS. (letter). *New England Journal of Medicine, 321,* 1408-1409.

Redfield, R.R., & Tramont, E.C. (Ed.) (1989). Toward a better classification system for HIV infection. *New England Journal of Medicine, 320,* 1414-1416.

Rhame, F.S. (Ed.) (1990). The HIV-infected surgeon. *Journal of the American Medical Association, 264,* 507-508.

Scitovsky, A.A., Cline, M., & Lee, P.R. (1986). Medical care costs of patients with AIDS in San Francisco. *Journal of the American Medical Association, 255,* 3103-3106.

Volberding, P. (1989). Supporting the health care team in caring for patients with AIDS. *Journal of the American Medical Association, 261,* 747-748.

Wachter, R.M., Luce, J.M., Hearst, N., & Lo, B. (1989). Decisions about resuscitation: inequities among patients with different diseases but similar prognosis. *Annals of Internal Medicine, 111,* 525-532.

The Staging and Monitoring by Primary Care Providers of Patients with Human Immunodeficiency Virus Infections

Michael A. Sauri

SUMMARY. As HIV testing expands through the population, primary care physicians will become more involved in the testing process. They will also be caring for increasingly larger numbers of HIV infected people from the asymptomatic through those with AIDS, through hospice care, should that become appropriate. This article summarizes key areas of clinician support for the HIV infected, clinical and laboratory markers associated with rapid progression of the disease, and important problem areas in clinical management. It also presents a series of staging diagrams that have proven useful in assisting clinicians in educating patients about the natural history of the HIV infection, the rationale for staging, the rationale for the timing of AZT therapy and Pneumocystis prophylactic treatment, and the significance of various prognosticators in management as the disease progresses.

INTRODUCTION

As HIV testing expands through the population, it is likely that primary care physicians will become more involved in the testing process. In addition, seropositive people will increasingly seek care

Michael A. Sauri, MD, MPH, TM, is an internist specializing in general internal medicine and clinical infectious diseases and tropical medicine. He is in private practice in the Washington, DC, metropolitan area. He is Assistant Professor in the Tropical Medicine Division of the Uniformed Services University of Health Sciences and a member of the Physician AIDS Advisory Committee of the Montgomery Hospice Society, Rockville, MD.

Address correspondence to the author at 9715 Medical Center Drive, Suite 201, Rockville, MD 20850.

and advice from primary care physicians. The majority of these people will be asymptomatic, some for several years. For this reason it will become essential for primary care physicians to learn as much as possible about the diagnosis, the staging, and the management of patients in all phases of this virally caused, degenerative disease characterized by progressive dysfunction of the immune system.

MAJOR AREAS OF SUPPORT AT THE PRIMARY CARE LEVEL FOR THE HIV INFECTED

Table 1 is a summary of the major areas of support that are delivered to HIV infected individuals at the primary care level.

Table 1

Key Areas of Support for HIV Infected

Patients at the Primary care Level

1.   Pre- and Post-test counseling

2.   Confidential/Anonymous HIV testing

3.   Initial Staging Work-up

4.   Prophylactic/Suppressive Management

5.   Nutritional assessment and management

6.   Source of Information

7.   Coordination of the patient's multi
     disciplinary care

8.   Clinical management

Testing

An accurate and detailed assessment of the risk of HIV infection must be made prior to confirming the clinical diagnosis with laboratory tests. HIV testing should be accomplished in conjunction with pre- and post-testing counseling. The patient should be offered the option of confidential versus anonymous testing. It should be emphasized that all medical records are considered confidential and are released only on written authorization of the patient. Anonymous testing means that in addition to the fact that a record of the testing or its results is not annotated in the patient's medical record, the results are known only to the patient through the use of an identification code number.

When the Diagnosis Has Been Established

After the diagnosis of HIV infection has been established, it is important, on the initial visit, to conduct a detailed review with the patient about the various aspects of HIV infection and AIDS. This should be accomplished with readily available, easy to comprehend patient teaching materials including handouts that the patient can take with him or her for later reference. Together with these handouts, a list of various points of contact with local information and support resources should be given to the patient. This will help to introduce her or him to the concept of continuity of care and provide early access to the multi-disciplinary community agencies involved in the management of HIV infection. It will also introduce the patient to the concepts of self-care and self-responsibility.

Counseling About Preventive Measures

The primary care physician should counsel about preventive measures such as "safe sex" and immunizations in order to reduce the spread of HIV infection, reduce the further "burden" of preventable infection and thereby reduce further destruction of the patient's immune system. Various immunizations are recommended due to the increased frequency of several preventable infections in asymptomatic and symptomatic HIV infected individuals. Immunizations for influenzae, hepatitis B, pneumococcus and Haemophilus influenzae have been recommended to all HIV patients. At the present time an AIDS vaccine to be given to uninfected people is not available to the public. Nevertheless, there are several experimental vaccines that are currently undergoing testing and may be available for general use in several years.

The Establishment of a Baseline Profile

The basic tests for an asymptomatic HIV-positive individual should establish a profile that can be used to monitor disease progression and it should establish data about prior exposure to pathogens that may subsequently reactivate as the immunosuppression progression increases. Initial screening tests that may be considered include complete blood count, platelet count, biochemistry profile including liver function tests, erythrocyte sedimentation rate, VDRL, hepatitis B antigen, an Anergy panel including a PPD skin test and a CD4 cell count.

Other tests to consider, depending on the stage of HIV disease progression and membership in a high risk group (Intravenous drug abusers, male homosexuals, etc.) include chest film, assays of antibodies to Toxoplasma, cytomegalovirus and Cryptococcus neoformans antigen. An examination of stool for enteric pathogens and ova and parasites should be considered due to the increased frequency of salmonella, helminthic, and protozoan infections in certain groups of HIV infected individuals.

Symptomatic Patients

For symptomatic patients, the severity of the disease is directly related to the degree of immune suppression in a continuous spectrum characterized by diverse and variable symptomatology. Thus we see that AIDS, rather than being a discreet clinical entity, is a set of case-defining infections or disorders that represent complications associated with an advanced stage of a chronic, progressive viral infection.

Staging as a Teaching Tool

As close to precise staging as possible of a patient with HIV infection is important for several reasons. First, it gives patients a realistic assessment of life expectancy. Second, it can help guide physicians as to how patients should be followed for the development of complications. Third, it provides data on which to base therapeutic decisions and parameters for measuring response to therapy. Fourth, specific staging of the diagnosis may entitle patients to increased assistance from local and federal governments. Finally, in satisfying FDA guidelines for determining eligibility for newly approved drugs/treatments (e.g., AZT, aerosolized pentamidine, erythropoietin, DHPG, etc.) we can assist patients with receiving reimbursement from private insurance.

In my practice I use a series of graphs to start to help the patient understand the natural history of the infection. I start out explaining the reason for the initial staging utilization, by using an adaptation of the Walter Reed Army Medical Center Staging Criteria for HIV Infection (see Figure One). I then superimpose a second graph depicting the timing of AZT therapy and Pneumocystis pneumonia prophylactic therapy (Figure Two). This provides an opportunity to emphasize the need for early therapy. Upon this I add a "slow track" and a "fast track" slope on either side of the "median track" of immune system failure and begin to explain the utility of various laboratory "prognosticators" (see Figure Three). This illustrates how the presence of various laboratory markers reflects the failure of the immune function.

The final product is a schematic that provides a basis of understanding for the patient of: (1) the natural history of HIV infection; (2) the rationale for staging; (3) the sequence of clinical disease from asymptomatic to opportunistic infections, through cancers due to the progressive destruction of the immune system; (4) the rationale for the use of and the timing of AZT therapy and Pneumocystis pneumonia prophylactic therapy; and (5) the significance of various prognosticators in the management of HIV infection (Figure Four).

Clinical and Laboratory Markers

With the exception of a few specific disease states for which survival data exist (i.e., the first or second episode of Pneumocystis carinii pneumonia, disseminated Mycobacterium avium intracellulare infection, or pulmonary Kaposi's sarcoma), clinical data alone cannot be relied on to assist in estimating prognosis. Table 2 sum-

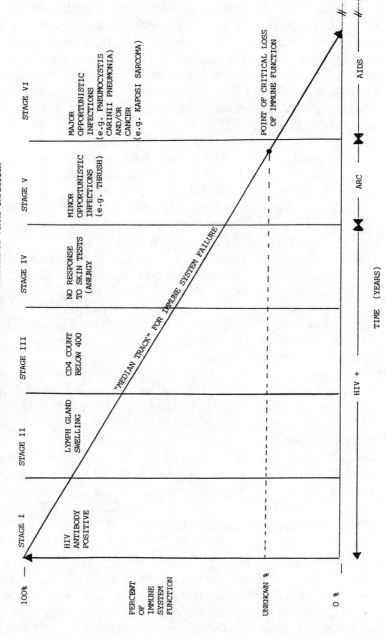

FIGURE ONE

NATURAL HISTORY OF HUMAN IMMUNODEFICIENCY VIRAL INFECTION

STAGE I	STAGE II	STAGE III	STAGE IV	STAGE V	STAGE VI
HIV ANTIBODY POSITIVE	LYMPH GLAND SWELLING	CD4 COUNT BELOW 400	NO RESPONSE TO SKIN TESTS (ANERGY	MINOR OPPORTUNISTIC INFECTIONS (e.g. THRUSH)	MAJOR OPPORTUNISTIC INFECTIONS (e.g. PNEUMOCYSTIS CARINII PNEUMONIA) AND/OR CANCER (e.g. KAPOSI SARCOMA)

"MEDIAN TRACK" FOR IMMUNE SYSTEM FAILURE

POINT OF CRITICAL LOSS OF IMMUNE FUNCTION

PERCENT OF IMMUNE SYSTEM FUNCTION

100%

UNKNOWN %

0 %

TIME (YEARS)

HIV +   ARC   AIDS

(Adapted from the Walter Reed Army Medical Center Staging Criteria for HIV Infection

18

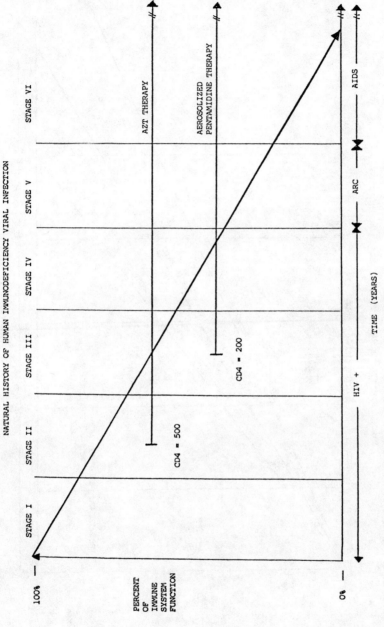

FIGURE TWO

NATURAL HISTORY OF HUMAN IMMUNODEFICIENCY VIRAL INFECTION

(Adapted from the Walter Reed Army Medical Center Staging Criteria for HIV Infection)

19

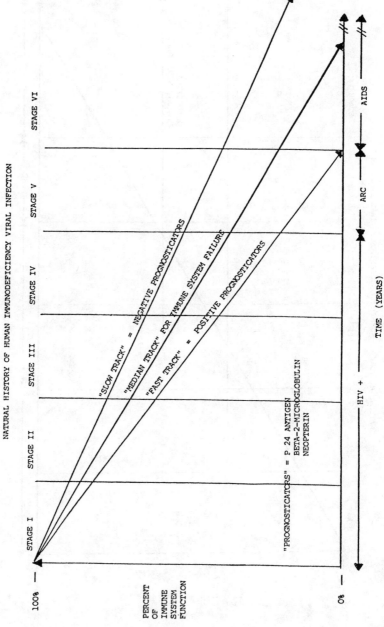

FIGURE THREE

NATURAL HISTORY OF HUMAN IMMUNODEFICIENCY VIRAL INFECTION

(Adapted from the Walter Reed Army Medical Center Staging Criteria for HIV Infection)

FIGURE FOUR

NATURAL HISTORY OF HUMAN IMMUNODEFICIENCY VIRAL INFECTION

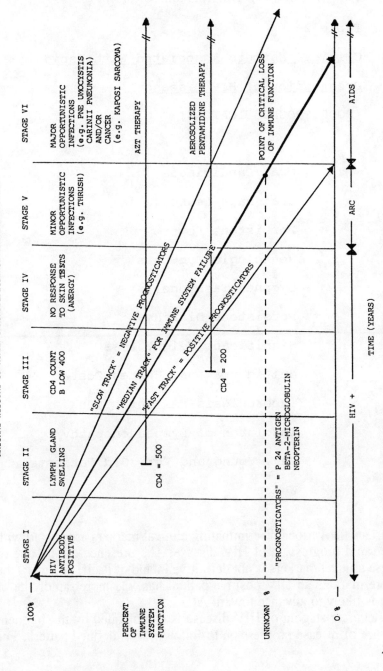

(Adapted from the Walter Reed Army Medical Center Staging Criteria for HIV Infection)

Table 2

Clinical Markers Associated With Rapid Progression of HIV Disease

(POOR PROGNOSTICATORS)

Oral Candidiasis

Oral hair Leukoplakia

Persistent Fever

Neurologic Symptoms

Dyspnea/Tachypnea

Persistent Diarrhea

Significant Weight Loss

Multidermatomal Herpes Zoster

Tuberculosis/MAI Infection

Involuton of Lymphadenopathy

Very Young and Very Old Patients

Women

marizes the various discriminating clinical markers associated with the rapid progression of HIV disease. The presence of any one of these clinical markers is not definitive in and of itself, however, the more markers an HIV positive patient has, the more rapidly he or she is likely to advance toward AIDS.

Accurate staging of HIV disease is complicated by the frequent failure of disease progression to follow a well-defined pattern. For example, a traditional view (Walter Reed Army Medical Center Staging Criteria [see Figure One]) may be represented by advancement from asymptomatic seropositivity to subclinical immune deficiency to lymphadenopathy to AIDS. It is not unusual, however, for a patient to progress from subclinical immune deficiency or lymphadenopathy rapidly and directly to an AIDS-defining opportunistic infection or condition.

Furthermore, clinical parameters are only useful in assessing symptomatic patients and not the majority of patients who are asymptomatic. As a result of this diversity in patient presentation and disease development, various laboratory markers must be used to supplement the clinical evaluation in order to identify those asymptomatic individuals in whom disease is otherwise rapidly advancing. Table 3 summarizes the laboratory markers that are associated with the rapid progression of HIV disease. The more laboratory markers that a patient has the more rapid the progression to AIDS. No individual laboratory marker is definitive by itself. Each must be viewed in the context of the overall clinical picture.

Prophylactic Management

Prophylactic management of HIV-infected patients consists of administering recommended immunizations such as influenzae, pneumococcal, hepatitis B and possibly Haemophilus Influenzae B vaccines. In addition, since the likelihood of Pneumocystis carinii pneumonia is high when the CD4 count falls below 200, initiation of prophylaxis with aerosolized pentamidine and other prophylactic agents has been shown to be effective. Positive PPD skin tests should be treated with 1-2 years of INH therapy. At present it is not clear that there is any effective prophylaxis against various other opportunistic infections (CMVV, toxoplasmosis, HSV, histoplasmosis, etc.). Since most of these infections are reactivations of prior infections or they reflect overgrowth of normal microflora, it may be more accurate to characterize the bulk of "prophylactic therapy" as simply suppressive therapy of chronic infections.

Table   3

Laboratory Markers Associated With the

Rapid Progression of HIV Disease

(POOR PROGNOSTICATORS)

Low or Declining Absolute CD4 Lymphocyte Count

    Or Percentage of CD4 Lymphocytes

Viremia

p24 Antigenemia

Decreased Antibody to p24 Antigen

Elevated Serum Beta-2-Microglobulin

Elevated Serum Neopterin

Anemia

Neutropenia

Thrombocytopenia

Persistent Anergy in Skin Testing

Serum Albumin less than 2 gms/dl

Hypoxemia less than 50 mmHg

Co-infection with Human T-cell Leukemia Virus

    (HTLV I and II)

Ongoing Nutritional Assessment

Nutritional assessment should be accomplished at the initial evaluation and repeated regularly. The best nutritional status should be maintained at all times. Poor nutrition contributes to the further suppression of cell-mediated immunity and reduces the number and efficacy of circulating lymphocytes. Due to intractable diarrheas, the increased metabolic rate of high fevers, and conditions in the mouth that may make eating or swallowing difficult, many HIV patients develop severe nutritional deficits. They are prone to dehydration and fluid volume depletion thus they may need intravenous rehydration and volume repletion at times. Patients should be monitored for the need for replenishment of electrolytes and tracemetals depleted by malnutrition (wasting syndrome) and by the adverse effects of various medications.

The administration of Megace has been found useful in counteracting the loss of appetite associated with HIV disease and its treatment. Not infrequently, entero-hyperalimentation and parenteral hyperalimentation is required to maintain the patient nutritionally during a period of treatment. The use of hyperalimentation is not contraindicated in HIV-infected patients, even those in hospice programs, and should not be discounted as a therapeutic option unless the patient has requested to forgo its use.

Other Aspects of the Role of the Primary Care Clinician

Information source. The patient views the primary care provider as the source of medical information, whether it is concerning the pros and cons of the most recent medical developments, the local resources involved in the multi-disciplinary and multi-agency approach to managing care, or the availability of his or her eligibility for relevant experimental protocols. At all times, the opportunity should be taken to counsel patients about newer therapies, their side effects, and their relationship to the disease process. Continuous monitoring is also suggested for evidence of self-medication with nonapproved agents or with approved agents not indicated for the patient's condition. In general, practitioners should not condemn these common attempts at self medication with "underground" remedies, but should keep current on these alternative therapies and should become aware of their potential effects in order to give appropriate advice.

Coordinator of care. The physician who is the primary care provider also serves as the coordinator for the patient within this multidisciplinary multi-agency approach. One patient's care may involve an array of medical specialists such as a dermatologist, an ophthalmologist, a gastroenterologist, a pulmonologist, an hematologist/ oncologist, a general surgeon, a radiation therapist, etc., as well as the involvement of hospice home care nurses, volunteers, psychiatric and family counseling, "buddy" groups, and transportation and shopping services. It may also include participation in protocols and Parallel Track drug trials.

Table 4 outlines the key problem areas in the clinical management of HIV infected patients. In the early stages of the infection, the patient is usually asymptomatic, the tone of the visits frequently upbeat, and the primary care physician is able to hold the frequency of visits and clinical evaluations to a minimum. In the more advanced stages of infection, the patient begins to exhibit the constellation of signs and symptoms incorporated in the AIDS-related complex (ARC) and AIDS, making it necessary for more frequent clinical and laboratory monitoring, and prophylaxis/suppressive therapy.

Although Table 4 does not address the more difficult challenge to the primary care professional of the various psychosocial aspects of HIV disease, it should be kept in mind that this is one area in which he or she should be most skillful in offering assistance. He or she should not only give time, active listening, and sensitive understanding, but should also be in touch with all community supports — financial as well as social and emotional — that can be brought to bear to sustain the best quality of life for patient and for family.

CONCLUSION

In the future, the majority of patients with HIV infection will come to the attention of primary care physicians. Through the process of staging, a determination of the patient's risk factors — symp-

Table 4. <u>Key Problem Areas in the</u>
<u>Clinical Management of HIV-infected Patients</u>

a. Retrovirus Infection Therapy

    1. AZT

    2. Parallel Track Therapies (ddI, etc.)

    3. "Underground"/Alternative Therapies

b. Management of Opportunistic Infection

    1. Cytomegalovirus Treatments

    2. Mycobacterium-avium-intracellulare
       Treatments

    3. Toxoplasmosis Treatment

    4. Herpes Simplex/Zoster Treatments

    5. Muco-cutaneous Candida Treatments

    6. Cryptococcal Infection Treatments

c. Management of Non-Opportunistic Infection
Complications

    1. Kaposi Sarcoma

    2. Lymphomas

    3. HIV Encephalopathy/neuropathy

Table 4 (continued)

d. Monitoring and Management of Drug-Related
    Complications
        1. Anemia due to:
                AZT therapy
                Ganciclovir therapy
                alpha interferon
                MAI infections
                tuberculosis
                cryptococcus
                histoplasmosis
        2. Neutropenia due to:
                AZT therapy
                Ganciclovir therapy
                DDI therapy
                Foscarnet therapy
        3. Nephrotoxicity due to:
                Pentamidine
                Aminoglycosides
                Vancomycin
                Amphotericin B

Flucytosie

4 . Hepatotoxicity due to:

Anti-TBC/MAI drugs

Ketoconazole/Fluconazole

5. Cytotoxicity due to:

Radiation therapy

Chemotherapeutic agents

6. Myositis due to:

AZT therapy

Sulfa drugs

7. Multi-drug interactions due to:

AZT + I.V. Bactrim

AZT + I.V. Pentamidine

AZT + I.V. Acyclovir

Ketoconazole + Zantac

8. Allergic Drug Reactions, due to:

Sulfa-containing agents

Dilantin

toms, clinical signs, laboratory predictors for rapid progression—is achieved. Familiarity with this process is essential for the primary care professional to properly advise the HIV infected patient about life expectancy, therapeutic options, and treatment responses.

The point at which hospice care becomes appropriate in the process of staging is determined by a complex of factors as the final stage is reached. These factors include the intersection of laboratory markers, clinical markers, and psycho-social-spiritual indicators.

BIBLIOGRAPHY OF USEFUL RESOURCES

Crocchiolo, P.R. et al. (1988). CD4 +; neopterin ratio significantly improves correlation with the Walter Reed Staging System if compared with CD4 + and neopterin considered separately. *AIDS, 2,* 481-2.

Diaz, J.D. et al. (1988). Classification systems for HIV infection. (Letter). *Annals of Internal Medicine, 108,* 155-6.

Haverkos, H.W. et al. (1985). Classification of HTLV III/LAV infection. (Letter). *Journal of Infectious Diseases, 152,* 1095.

Justice, A.C et al. (1989). A new prognostic staging system for AIDS. *New England Journal of Medicine, 320,* 1388-1393.

Miles, S.A. (1988). Diagnosis and staging of HIV infection. *American Family Physician, 38,* 248-56.

MMWR (1986). Classification system for HTLV-III/Lymphadenopathy-associated virus infection. *35,* 334-339.

MMWR (1987). Classification system for HIV infection in children under 13 years of age. *36,* 225-230.

MMWR (1988). Revision of HIV classification codes. *36,* Supplement 1S.

Moss, A.R. et al. (1988). Seropositivity for HIV and the development of AIDS and AIDS related condition: three year follow up of the San Francisco General Hospital Cohort. *British Medical Journal (Clinical Research), 296,* (6624) 745-50.

Principi, N. et al. (1988). Problems of classification of HIV-seropositive pediatric patients. *Pediatric Infectious Diseases Journal, 7,* 466-468.

Redfield, R.R., Wright, D.C., & Tramont E.D. (1986). The Walter Reed Staging Classification of HTLV-III infection. *New England Journal of Medicine, 314,* 131-132.

Redfield, R.R., & Tramont, E.C. (1989). Toward a better classification system for HIV infection. *New England Journal of Medicine, 320,* 1414-6.

Rogers, M.F., & Curran, J.W. (1988). Problems of classification of HIV-seropositive pediatric patients. *Pediatric Infectious Diseases Journal,* (Letter) *7,* 889-890.

Solomon, S.L., & Curran, J.W. (1987). Public health applications of a classification system for HIV infection. *Annals of Internal Medicine, 106,* 319-20.

Turner, B.J. et al. (1989). A severity classification system for AIDS hospitalizations. *Medical Care, 17,* 423-37.

Yarchoan, R., & Pluda, J.M. (1988). Clinical aspects of infection with AIDS retrovirus: Acute HIV infection, persistent generalized lymphadenopathy, and AIDS-Related complex. Chapter 7 in DeVita, V.T., Hellman, S., & Rosenberg, S.A. (Eds.) *AIDS: Etiology, Diagnosis, Treatment, and Prevention* (2nd ed.). Philadelphia: J.B. Lippincott Co.

Issues in the Current Treatment
of Hospice Patients with HIV Disease

Jeannee Parker Martin

SUMMARY. Hospice administrators and clinicians face many complex issues regarding the treatment of persons terminally ill with AIDS, at one end of the spectrum of HIV disease. Among these issues are: whether the hospice model applies to persons with AIDS; at what point does the person with AIDS receive palliative rather than curative therapy; and what alternatives exist for hospice care if the AIDS patient has no primary care provider or no home in which to receive care. This article delineates and discusses these issues.

INTRODUCTION

The term HIV disease is used throughout this article to denote a spectrum of illness. At one end are persons with HIV infection who are asymptomatic. They do not yet have AIDS or an AIDS qualify-

Jeannee Parker Martin, RN, MPH, has been involved in the care of persons with HIV disease since 1982. She has been the Executive Director, Hospice Programs of the Visiting Nurses and Hospice of San Francisco since 1986. Ms. Martin has represented home and hospice care issues in the care of persons with HIV disease on many local, state and national advisory councils. She has testified before the Presidential Commission on HIV Disease and served as a consultant to the World Health Organization on the out-of-hospital care of persons with HIV disease. In addition, she has lectured, consulted and written extensively on other issues related to home care, hospice care, and HIV disease.

The author thanks Robert V. Brody, MD, Medical Director for the Hospice Programs of Visiting Nurses and Hospice of San Francisco and internist at San Francisco General Hospital; Christine Cody, RN, CMSN, Assistant Director, Hospice Programs; Anne M. Hughes, RN, MN, CFNP, AIDS Clinical Nurse Specialist at San Francisco General Hospital; and Marylin Dodd, RN, PhD, FAAN, Professor and Interim Chair of the Department of Physiological Nursing, University of California at San Francisco.

Address correspondence to the author at Visiting Nurses and Hospice of San Francisco, Fox Plaza, 1390 Market St., Suite 510, San Francisco, CA 94102.

ing condition but they are likely to progress to AIDS at some point. Persons with symptomatic HIV disease are those infected with the virus who have early symptoms such as thrush, skin infections, chronic fatigue, diarrhea, or generalized lymphadenopathy but lack a diagnosed opportunistic infection or cancer, the markers of an AIDS diagnosis. The spectrum of care for these people has been described as a response to a continuum of disability (Schietinger, 1986). The continuum comprises four interrelated though not necessarily sequential stages. Those:

1. apparently well with asymptomatic HIV disease
2. acutely ill with symptomatic HIV disease or AIDS
3. chronically ill with symptomatic HIV disease or AIDS
4. terminally ill with AIDS

Countless numbers of people in the United States are infected with HIV and may live active, relatively symptom free lives for many years. According to a recent study the median incubation period from the time of infection with HIV to diagnosis with AIDS in homosexual men is approximately 11.0 years (Lemp, 1990). During this period if the HIV infected develop early symptoms they may want treatment or, in the hope of staving off more severe symptoms, they may seek prophylactic measures. Once diagnosed with one of the several opportunistic infections and/or secondary cancers characteristic of AIDS, however, life expectancy becomes short—approximately 18 months.

Some experts have estimated that approximately 5% of persons diagnosed with AIDS will require the sensitive and patient/family-centered approach of hospice care. In the 1990s all hospice providers must be prepared to address the complex physical, psychosocial, spiritual, and bereavement needs of persons with AIDS. Like their patients, hospice providers will be challenged to understand the complexities of this illness and its constantly evolving new treatments. Hospice programs, in addition, will be asked to provide guidance and support to persons with AIDS who are referred for services and/or to grieving family members whose son or daughter has died of AIDS in a distant place.

APPLYING THE HOSPICE MODEL
TO PERSONS WITH AIDS

Perhaps one of the most difficult dilemmas hospice providers face is determining when or if hospice care applies to persons with AIDS.

The hospice philosophy of care is intended to provide physical, psychosocial, and spiritual comfort to persons in the last stages of incurable disease who have chosen a palliative rather than a curative approach to care. Furthermore, this approach provides emotional support and guidance to members of the family, however defined, prior to the death of the loved one and during the subsequent period of bereavement (Hall & Kirschling, 1990). Focusing on the patient and family as the unit of care, the hospice model allows the patient to live with dignity during the final days, weeks, or months of life and most often in the comfortable and familiar surroundings of home.

According to this definition hospice care aptly applies to the care of persons terminally ill with AIDS. However, even among the most experienced hospice caregivers, AIDS provokes intense debate about which treatments are curative and which are palliative. At what point is the patient terminally ill or in the last stages of incurable disease? Is prophylactic therapy for Pneumocystis carinii pneumonia or long term ganciclovir (DHPG) infusion for cytomegalovirus (CMV) appropriate when the patient has only a short time to live? These therapies may be needed indefinitely and may require frequent nursing visits for medication administration. Who makes treatment decisions if the patient is unable to do so and there is no properly designated surrogate decision maker? A dimension that frequently confounds the discussion further is who should pay for costly medications or treatments that may palliate symptoms without curing the underlying HIV infection?

Hospice Eligibility Criteria

These concerns are even more provocative to hospice provider programs that have limiting eligibility criteria, for example, those that restrict admissions to cancer patients, to those with clearly identifiable primary care providers, to those enrolled in particular insurance programs, or to those that do not require intravenous therapies. Most hospice programs carefully select the eligibility criteria that best meet the needs of their service area, financial capabilities, and the skills of their staff and volunteers. Modifications in eligibility criteria may require governing board approval and careful discussion with staff and volunteers at all levels. Whatever the restrictions, they should not be considered barriers to persons with AIDS specifically, but rather barriers to any terminally ill patient not meeting the conditions.

To properly discern whether its philosophy does apply to an individual disease entity, each hospice program should first examine its mission. Does the agency's philosophy encompass the precepts described above? Are there inherent limitations restricting care to certain groups, for example only cancer patients? Has the hospice provider considered modifying its mission to include previously unserved groups?

After a review of the mission, the hospice program should review its eligibility criteria. Do they limit the agency to serving particular patients? Are there restrictions based on insurance coverage or other reimbursement sources? Does the hospice program accept patients receiving intravenous therapy or provide such services if a patient requires palliative intravenous therapy for pain or symptom management? If the hospice program adheres to an admission criterion of a diagnosis of cancer, does it admit persons with AIDS with Kaposi's sarcoma or primary lymphoma of the brain?

There is no "correct" answer to any of these questions. One expert program may believe in restrictions; another in as few limitations as possible. Whatever the answers, however, AIDS as a diagnosis should not be a barrier to hospice admission. A person with AIDS should be considered fairly and treated in a manner consistent with all other eligible patients if he or she meets the eligibility criteria for the hospice program.

Given the above considerations, then, the hospice philosophy does, in fact, apply to many diagnosed with AIDS. It clearly applies to patients: (1) who are in the last phases of their disease (sometimes defined as a disease prognosis of six months or less); (2) who have chosen palliative care and no longer seek a cure for their disease (or, if unable to choose due to mental status impairment, their designated surrogate decision maker may assist with the decision for palliative therapy); (3) who have a designated primary care provider, or a supportive caregiving network, or who have accepted institutionalization should their home environment become inappropriate for their continued care (e.g., they need continuous care due to physical and mental status debilitation); and, (4) who have accepted hospice care and understand the limitations imposed by a particular program (e.g., if intravenous fluids are required for palliative care, other arrangements may need to be made for its administration).

Indicators of the Terminal Phase of HIV Disease

There are no absolute indicators for demarcating the terminal phase of HIV disease. Experience, however, has offered some clues as to when a person may be in the last stages. In addition, many hospice providers are experienced in determining life expectancy and they should be able to apply these same skills to persons with AIDS.

Indicators that may be helpful in determining whether a patient is in the terminal phase of HIV illness may include the following considerations. These will generally be patients who have been diagnosed with AIDS for many months and whose physical status is deteriorating. They usually have had increasingly frequent episodes of opportunistic infections, such as three or four bouts of Pneumocystis carinii pneumonia, cryptosporidiosis, or CMV. They may have dissemination of neoplasms, such as Kaposi's sarcoma or non-Hodgkin's lymphoma. Additional indicators may be severe wasting syndrome, progressive decline of mental status, generalized deterioration of all body systems, and unresponsiveness to treatment.

Palliative versus Curative Therapy

The hospice philosophy of relieving pain and untoward symptoms rather than curing the underlying disease is simultaneously appropriate for the care of persons with AIDS and in conflict with the goals of many of these patients and their families or caregivers. Who makes the decision as to what is palliative and what is curative: the patient and family? the physician? the nurse? the reimbursement source? the scientist/researcher? the hospice interdisciplinary team?

It is well known that presently there is no cure for the HIV infection which causes AIDS. It is also known that, other than zidovudine (AZT), which has antiviral properties and increases the time before there is an onset of more severe symptoms in some infected individuals, and perhaps its analogs, dideoxynosine (ddi) and dideoxycytidine (ddc) there is no treatment currently available to cure HIV disease. The interventions currently available to treat the opportunistic infections and neoplasms associated with AIDS generally offer temporary symptomatic relief and often must be continued indefinitely to assure continued relief. Although difficult for many patients and their families or caregivers to accept, most available medications, even those for the minor infections associated with HIV disease, are truly palliative rather than curative.

Most persons with AIDS take many medications and receive treatments for opportunistic infections until they are physically unable to continue them. This practice may be confusing to traditional hospice caregivers, since many of these medications may appear to have no effect on symptoms or at best they may only provide minor relief. Patients and family members, however, may be reluctant to terminate even minor medications for fear the disease will progress more rapidly or be more severe.

Intravenous Therapy

Another frequent discussion is whether intravenous therapies, particularly for total parental nutrition (TPN), are appropriate to administer if the patient chooses hospice care. The goal of such therapy should be considered before the decision to institute it is made. Goals in hospice care may include short term treatment to determine if an infection can be brought under control or palliation of particular symptoms. Hospice care goals may also include the attainment of a personal goal such as the arrival of a loved one, or a birthday, or time to legally complete a will. For example, if the patient has an opportunistic infection or sequelae, intravenous medication is often appropriate to minimize further symptoms. If the therapy is not relieving symptoms, then it should be discontinued.

The goal of any intravenous therapy should be reviewed frequently. Although the experienced hospice clinician in all likelihood would not typically advocate the use of TPN in terminally ill patients, such therapy may temporarily promote the physical and emotional well-being of both the patient and the family. TPN or hydration should not be considered for long term maintenance in any terminally ill patient. The risks and costs far outweigh the benefits.

When the Person with AIDS Does Not Want to Give Up Hope of Cure

Returning, then, to the premise that the hospice philosophy focuses on palliative therapy and that most of the treatment persons with AIDS receive is truly palliative, persons with AIDS should fit neatly into the missions of most hospice care programs. However, many persons with AIDS, despite severe and debilitating illness, continue to dream of an imminent cure. They live on the hope that they will be the first ones to survive, that just one more treatment or new therapy will bring back their immune function.

Hospice teams have extensive familiarity with this attitude. In their practices they see many patients with untreatable cancer who are not ready to accept the inevitable at the time of admission to the hospice. Often the patient has been encouraged by a friend or family member or physician to seek hospice care. In all these cases, it is the hospice interdisciplinary team that guides and supports these uncertain or ambivalent patients as they gradually come to terms with their prognoses. Persons with AIDS are no different and should be encouraged to participate in a hospice program of care. Once in hospice, however, these patients should not be discouraged from continuing a particular treatment regime if it is successful in alleviating physical or emotional symptoms.

When the Patient Has No Primary Care Provider

Many hospice providers limit admissions to patients with primary care providers. Usually primary care providers are family members who live with the patient and/or are available 24 hours a day to assist the patient should physical or mental deterioration occur. Unlike other hospice patients, persons with AIDS often live alone or have a partner who works and/or may have HIV disease as well. In the absence of an available primary care provider, AIDS patients are usually unable to pay out-of-pocket fees for costly attendant care to supply the necessary personal care and supervision as their disease progresses. In addition, persons with AIDS often become medically indigent due to expenditures of financial resources for costly treatments and medications or the loss of health insurance after they are unable to work. These dynamics can severely compromise the capacity of an agency to provide hospice care.

Care Settings Outside the Home

In the absence of primary care providers and adequate financial resources to pay for surrogate caregivers, some hospice programs have turned to alternative settings outside the home. These alternatives may include adult day health care or social day care centers, skilled nursing facilities, or group residential housing arrangements.

Adult day health or social day care centers allow the patient to receive supervision and care in a structured environment for approximately 8 hours each day while the primary caregivers are at work. These centers are generally licensed by state agencies and are eligible for reimbursement under public and private insurance programs. Attendees, brought to the center with sponsored transportation services, can participate in therapeutic activities throughout the day, and are able to socialize with other participants.

Skilled nursing facilities may be a limited option for patients with continuous care needs. Unfortunately, few communities have skilled nursing facilities that will accommodate AIDS patients due to age restrictions and limited bed capacities.

An appealing option to many hospice providers has been the development of group housing arrangements. These group houses or congregate residential facilities allow patients to benefit from the interdisciplinary hospice approach while at the same time spreading the costs of maintaining a private residence and by providing attendant care. Additional economies of scale may be derived by assigning hospice nurses and social workers to one group house, thus decreasing the time and cost of transportation.

Although this option may not be available in many communities it is a model of cost-effectiveness to consider and an option that has been looked on favorably by private and public grantmakers. Operationally, group houses are often maintained by an agency other than the hospice care provider. This allows the facility operator to access moneys pertinent to room and board charges while the hospice provider bills the patient's public or private reimbursement source. (For detailed information regarding the development of residential facilities for persons with HIV see: Haskell, Satten, Franks, and Martin (Eds). *Developing AIDS Residential Settings: A Manual (1988)*. San Francisco: Visiting Nurses and Hospice of San Francisco.)

CONCLUSION

Hospice providers will be challenged further by the demands of caring for persons with HIV disease. Agencies must examine their missions to assure that they are applied equally to all terminally ill patients. They must also review their eligibility criteria to determine what barriers, if any, may limit access to care for persons with HIV disease. If the widely accepted hospice philosophy is adopted, there will be few real barriers to the care of persons with HIV disease.

Some patients will be unwilling to accept their disease prognosis and others may want to pursue aggressive, curative therapy. Yet other patients will need surrogate caregivers if hospice care is to become a reality for them. All hospice programs should be prepared, however, to accept referrals for persons with HIV disease who meet the hospice's eligibility criteria and who accept limitations should the circumstances of their care require change.

REFERENCES

Hall, J.E., & Kirschling, J.M. (1990). A conceptual framework for caring for families of hospice patients. *The Hospice Journal, 6*(2), 1-28.

Haskell, W., Satten, N., Franks, P., & Martin, J. (Eds.) (1988). *Developing AIDS Residential Settings: A Manual*. San Francisco: Visiting Nurses and Hospice of San Francisco.

Lemp, G.F., Payne, S.F., Rutherford, G.W. et al. (1990). Projections of AIDS morbidity and mortality in San Francisco. *Journal of the American Medical Association, 263,* 1497-1501.

Schietinger H. (1986). A home care plan for AIDS. *American Journal of Nursing, 35,* 655-66.

The Cost of Caring for Patients with HIV Infection in Hospice

Claire Tehan

SUMMARY. This article explores the organizational barriers that have limited the number of persons with AIDS cared for by hospice programs throughout the United States. The financial implications of caring for persons with AIDS are discussed and data from a survey of 15 hospice providers is presented. Examples of creative and cooperative coalitions among hospice programs and other community organizations that maximize scarce resources and share the financial burden of caring for those infected with HIV are presented as models. The diverse funding sources and individual hospice program decisions about palliative treatments and drugs and admission criteria highlight the difficulty of generalizing from the survey.

Claire Tehan, MA, is presently Vice President for Hospice at Hospital Home Health Care Agency of California, a post she has held since 1977, Chair of the National Hospice Organization AIDS Resource Committee, and President of the California State Hospice Association. She has been active in the American hospice movement since 1975 and has served six years on the National Hospice Organization Board of Directors.

For their contributions the author thanks Mary Cook of Cabrini Hospice, Carolyn Fitzpatrick-Cassin of Hospice of Southeast Michigan, Bruce Fortin of Home Hospice of Sonoma, Sarah Gorodezky of Kaiser Permanente-Oakland, Rebecca McDonald of Hospice of Volusia-Flagler, Peter Moberg-Sarver of Hospice of Central New York, Jeannee Parker Martin of Visiting Nurses and Hospice of San Francisco, Carole Selinske of the New York State Hospice Association, Jo Ann Siemsen of Hospice Caring Project, Bill Wallace of the Hospice at Mission Hill, Cristy Whitney of Hospice of Northern Virginia, and Fran Zonfrillo of the Visiting Nurse Association of Los Angeles.

Address correspondence to the author c/o Hospital Home Health Care, 2061 Airport Drive #110, Torrance, CA 90505.

INTRODUCTION

That AIDS is a terminal illness is now well accepted. Since the disease was identified in 1981, the Centers for Disease Control (CDC) has reported 152,231 people diagnosed of whom 92,375 or 62% have died (CDC, 1990).

Looking at the data collected by the National Hospice Organization (NHO) about persons with AIDS cared for by hospices throughout the United States, it might seem that a very small proportion of them have received hospice care. In 1988, hospices responding to an NHO survey reported caring for 6,713 AIDS patients and in 1989, 8,048 (NHO 1988; NHO, 1989).

There are many reasons why the number of persons with AIDS cared for by hospices in the United States would appear to be low. Although concern over the financial burden is the focus of this article, we will also review other major deterrents to hospice care for this population.

NON-COST BARRIERS TO HOSPICE CARE FOR PERSONS WITH AIDS

Patient Barriers

Patient barriers are those factors that preclude a person with AIDS from choosing hospice care. One of the most obvious is age. Most persons with AIDS are young and not ready to accept a rapidly advancing incurable disease. In fact, since the onset of the epidemic in the gay community the emphasis has been to fight the disease; to not give up just because one is diagnosed. This determination and optimism resulted initially in the nationwide mobilization of action against the disease by the gay community. The ensuing political pressure produced the release of experimental drugs and an increase in funding for research and treatment, as well as the development of comprehensive and specialized services for persons with AIDS.

Hospice care, with its focus on acceptance of death and delivery of palliative and supportive care, was largely viewed by the gay community as inappropriate for AIDS patients. To these people hospice care represented, and to a considerable degree still does represent, an admission of failure—failure in that the disease becomes the acknowledged victor. It has been difficult to communicate the positive aspect central to the hospice philosophy that supports their fighting spirit—the concept of the empowerment of the individual.

The epidemic has changed, however, since 1984 and thanks to drugs such as AZT, pentamidine isothionate, and DHPG, patients who once would have died within months of developing AIDS, can now expect to live for well over a year. It appears that AIDS is becoming a chronic illness with a more clearly defined terminal phase. This will make it easier to determine when hospice care becomes appropriate.

Organizational Barriers

Many other barriers to hospice care for persons with AIDS are organizational. Hospice programs in the United States evolved primarily as a response to the physical, emotional, psychological, and spiritual needs of terminally ill cancer patients. Admission criteria, program components, and reimbursement applied to a primarily elderly population that most often included an intact and organized family support system.

Traditional hospice admission criteria include a prognosis of six months or less, forgoing of curative measures, emphasis on palliative and supportive care, and availability of a primary caregiver. Fitting the average AIDS patient into these criteria is like forcing a square peg into a round hole.

Prognosis. In the early years of the AIDS epidemic, the relatively few physicians who were caring for AIDS patients were often unable to predict with any certainty the progression of the disease, let alone prognosis. Many were also unwilling to confront the issue of terminality with their patients. Since hospice criteria generally require the physician to certify in writing that the patient has a prognosis of six months or less, hospice care was rarely considered by either the AIDS patient or his physician as a desirable option. Early on the Visiting Nurses and Hospice of San Francisco developed a less rigorous admissions policy that specified limited prognosis and a need for skilled nursing care in the home. This policy accommodated the AIDS patient's need to continue treatments that might be considered curative while simultaneously seeking the comfort and support of hospice care (Beresford, 1989).

Palliative Care. Another organizational barrier was and remains the hospice emphasis on only palliative and supportive care. Traditionally, the assumption has been that a cancer patient is referred to hospice after surgery, radiation, and/or chemotherapy treatments have been completed and there is no further curative treatment feasible. At that point, pain and symptom management and psychosocial support are all directed toward comfort.

AIDS is still a new disease with continually emerging treatments. There is little agreement about what constitutes curative and what constitutes palliative care. What is aggressive treatment for AIDS? Is AZT, relieving symptoms and extending life for a short time, palliative? Should aerosol pentamidine isothionate and DHPG, prophylactic drugs that prevent pneumonia and CMV retinitis respectively, be considered palliative or curative? There is as yet no accepted standard. Each hospice decides what is within the scope of its particular program. Physicians and persons with AIDS view this uncertainty as a limitation of their options.

Primary Caregiver. The third traditional requirement for hospice admission that served as a barrier has been that each patient must have a primary caregiver who assumes responsibility for either directly providing or coordinating the patient's care. This does not require the presence of the primary caregiver in the patient's home 24-hours a day. It does mean, however, that this person must make provision for such coverage if the patient's condition demands it.

Although this requirement is reasonable from the hospice's perspective, it is not practical for large numbers of persons with AIDS who wish to remain in their own homes. There may be family, lovers, and friends who want to help, but often their availability is limited. They cannot meet the needs of a patient who is too weak to lift his head off the pillow. In such cases attendant care is needed around the clock.

There are vast numbers of persons with AIDS who have no primary support at all. They have been abandoned by friends and family. These people are, a priori, precluded from considering hospice care if the program has a primary caregiver requirement.

These three admission criteria have been significant deterrents to hospice care for persons with AIDS. It is the attitude of many programs that if they modify these criteria to accommodate AIDS patients, they will be redefining hospice care for all terminally ill patients. Other programs do not believe they have the resource capability of meeting the needs of persons with AIDS if they alter the admission criteria. If the primary caregiver requirement is eliminated, it becomes the hospice's responsibility to provide for the patient's safety and care on a 24-hour basis. If palliative care is more broadly defined, the so called high-tech treatment needs of patients must be provided for or arranged by the hospice.

Current Cost Barriers to Hospice Care
for Persons with AIDS

The financial issues related to caring for persons with AIDS are an additional barrier to hospice care. Third party reimbursement is generally inadequate, especially given the high number of Medicaid covered and medically indigent AIDS patients. Although hospice programs express willingness to care for persons with AIDS, many are concerned about the financial burden of doing so. This concern is legitimate and it is the primary purpose of this article to present some of the creative strategies developed by hospice programs as a response to the financial challenges of the AIDS epidemic.

First, however, let us examine the existing reimbursement system in order to understand the fiscal constraints.

THE SURVEY

Since review of the literature in the Fall of 1990 revealed no recent data on the costs of caring for persons with AIDS at home, we conducted a national telephone survey of hospice providers experienced in AIDS care. We asked about the number of AIDS patients cared for in the previous year, the composition of that population (i.e., homosexual, IV drug user, women, children), and payer source. We also sought data on the program's average number of visits per AIDS patient, costs per day and/or costs per patient length of stay, as well as the cost per day of drugs, attendants, supplies, and equipment. In addition, we asked specific questions about Medicaid reimbursement and/or special state program funding.

A major shortcoming of the survey was that it was difficult to compare the data in that each program collected its statistics in a slightly different format. In addition, those hospice programs able to access funding for attendant care showed extremely high costs for attendants; other programs with no such funding were limited in what they could offer, therefore in what they could document. Although the survey highlighted the need to standardize data collection in order to obtain a truer picture of the costs of caring for persons with AIDS, trends and observations did emerge that can be valuable for program planning.

Table 1, in particular, illustrates the proportional payer distribution for AIDS patients receiving hospice care.

Medicaid

The experience of these hospices was that the proportion of Medicaid and medically indigent AIDS patients was extremely high. In most traditional hospice programs Medicaid patients account for only 10%-20% of the entire caseload. A high percentage of Medicaid reimbursed patients in a hospice program can have very serious financial implications.

Reimbursement under fee for service Medicaid in most parts of the country is generally well below the cost of providing that care. In California, an RN visit is reimbursed at $63.60; an MSW visit at $81.75. Costs for hospice programs in California, however, average $110.00 for an RN visit and $120.00 for an MSW visit. In Connecticut, Medicaid will not reimburse for a social worker or dietary consultant, two professionals very important to the care of persons with AIDS.

As a major payer of care for persons with AIDS, the Medicaid system is hampered by being a large bureaucracy with too few dollars to meet the health care needs of a state's poor. In California Medicaid has run out of money for the last two years. As a result, court ordered emergency payments were made to skilled nursing facilities, the only health care providers who received Medicaid re-

Table 1.
Proportional Payer Distribution for AIDS Patients
in Eight Hospices

HOSPICE	MEDICAID Percent	MEDICARE Percent	PRIVATE (Incl. HMO) Percent	MEDICALLY INDIGENT Percent
Hospice of Southeast Michigan Southfield, MI	71	< 1	14	14
Hospice of Northern Virginia Arlington, VA	11	14	64	11 *
Mission Hill Hospice Boston, MA	61	8	30	< 1
Hospital Home Health Care Agency of California Torrance, CA	47	3	39	10
VNA of Los Angeles Los Angeles, CA	39	3	31	27 **
Hospice of Volusia-Flagler Daytona Beach, FL	83	8	< 1	8
Visiting Nurses and Hospice of San Francisco San Francisco, CA	50	14.5	35.5	0
The Connecticut Hospice Branford, CT	80	0	10	10

*   Patients with CHAMPUS which does not cover Hospice care.

** Patients whose care is covered by L.A. County AIDS Funding

imbursement in the final month of the 1989-90 Fiscal Year. This uncertainty of payment, even when care is authorized, is an undeniable disincentive for programs faced with the care of large numbers of Medicaid patients.

The Medicaid Hospice Benefit

The Medicaid Hospice Benefit offered in 26 states was modeled on the Medicare Hospice Benefit, with the rates based on hospice experience with cancer patients. The range and volume of services required for a person with AIDS, including extensive attendant care and costly drugs, means increased costs in providing hospice care under the Medicaid Benefit.

The Home and Community-Based Waiver Program

The Home and Community-Based Waiver Program offered in eight states — California, Hawaii, Illinois, Ohio, New Jersey, Florida, North Carolina, and South Carolina — enables providers to offer additional services beyond those the state Medicaid program covers. Home health aides, homemakers, adult day care, skilled nursing, and medications are a few examples of services a hospice program could offer AIDS patients (Contreras, 1990). In the state of New York, Medicaid coverage for persons with AIDS is extremely generous; in fact, the availability of 24-hour attendant care through the AIDS Waiver Program far exceeds what a Medicare/Medicaid certified hospice can provide. Thus, the Visiting Nurse Service of New York City cares for most AIDS patients through their AIDS Home Care Program and very few through their basic hospice program. In Massachusetts, the Visiting Nurse Association of Boston is generously funded by the state to provide home care to persons with AIDS. Local Medicare/Medicaid certified hospices are unable to compete with the extensive services available through the VNA program. In other states Medicaid programs have made it easier to provide the appropriate level of care through pilot projects, special funding, or Home and Community-Based Waiver programs.

Alternatives

Although there is no escaping the reality of risk in caring for persons with AIDS under a fixed rate per diem reimbursement scheme, there are options and opportunities that can be explored. The New York State Hospice Association was successful in establishing a supplemental financial assistance program to cover the increased costs of caring for persons with special needs, in this case, persons with AIDS. The State Association introduced legislation that amended the public health law to pay hospices an additional amount of money to care for persons with special needs. On July 1, 1990, Medicare/Medicaid certified hospices in New York

City began receiving $164.56/day to care for persons with AIDS compared to $94.97 for Routine Home Care to other hospice patients. Hospice programs in Syracuse now receive $172.90/day for persons with AIDS compared to $99.66 for Routine Home Care. An escort rate is also included to pay for the additional cost of providing security for hospice staff. The increased rates are adjusted for SMSA areas throughout the state and include each of the levels of care paid for by the Hospice Medicare/Medicaid Benefit.

In Michigan, hospice leaders persuaded the state legislature to approve a schedule of drugs, including AZT, to be paid for outside of the Hospice Medicaid Benefit.

These successes in improving hospice reimbursement for persons with AIDS were the result of concerted efforts by state associations representing hospice care providers that had good reputations and track records in the provision of quality care. In New York there was precedence for supplemental funding for people with special needs and the emphasis on home care represents a huge financial saving to a system already overwhelmed by the cost of inpatient care.

Attendant Care in the Home

The most consistent finding among hospice providers in our sample was that the need for attendant care among persons with AIDS is very high. If a patient is going to remain at home, the need for this service should be anticipated. At the Visiting Nurses and Hospice of San Francisco, which has received substantial funding from the city for attendant care, AIDS patients used it an average of six hours/day.

The County of Los Angeles funds attendant care for AIDS patients receiving home care services. As a result, the Visiting Nurse Association of Los Angeles can provide an average of 90 hours a month per patient.

Since the need for attendant care is so great, hospice providers should consider taking a proactive position in seeking specific funding. A strong case can be made to local community and church groups about the cost savings as well as the humane value of assisting a person to remain at home. The director of Hospice of Volusia-

Flagler in Daytona Beach, Florida, obtained a Medicaid Home and Community-Based Waiver which allows her a supplemental $1000 per month per patient to be spent on such nontraditional Florida Medicaid services as home health aides and attendants. Several other hospices have received funding from private foundations for primary caregivers for those patients who would otherwise be ineligible for hospice care.

In Los Angeles, Hospital Home Health Care Agency of California has developed working relationships with three separate community organizations that manage residential group homes. The attendants, employed by the homes, are not the financial responsibility of the hospice program. When there are patients with heavy personal care needs, the hospice provides its own home health aides.

Prescription Drugs

There are several important issues when we consider the costs of providing prescription drugs under the Hospice Medicaid Benefit. Which drugs are considered palliative, thus paid for under the Hospice Medicaid Benefit? Several hospices have made the determination that AZT is not appropriate for AIDS patients receiving hospice care because it is not symptom-specific. Others have deemed it acceptable.

To make a decision about which medications and procedures are appropriate for persons with AIDS contingent on who is paying the bill can leave a hospice program open to charges of discrimination. These decisions admittedly difficult, should reflect the philosophy of the particular agency. Hospice programs in San Francisco and Santa Cruz, California and in Miami, Florida have modified the parameters of their programs by expanding their services. They have liberally defined palliative care, with resulting success in serving significant numbers of persons with AIDS.

In Los Angeles, two major hospice providers, Hospital Home Health Care Agency of California and the Visiting Nurse Association of Los Angeles, collaborated in the development of a formulary of reimbursable drugs. This was a valuable process. Although initially there was considerable difference of opinion, in the end there was consensus. Each program, after internal review, subsequently adopted the formulary. Having the formulary has precluded patients and/or physicians in the area from playing one program against the other on the basis of drug benefits.

In our national survey we found no consistency among providers as to a standard formulary, thus an average cost per day for drugs could not readily be calculated. On gross analysis, however, some distinctions emerged. Those programs paying for AZT, amphotericin, and aerosol pentamidine isothionate claimed an average cost of from $27.00 to $55.00 a day for drugs. For programs that generally did not cover those medications, the average daily cost ranged from $17.00 to $36.00.

Professional Services

Our survey revealed no consensus among hospice executives that persons with AIDS consistently require more visits from hospice professionals. There was wide variation in experience reported with some patients receiving daily RN visits for the administration of IV therapies and others needing RN visits only twice a week. At Hospital Home Health Care Agency of California as staff became more experienced, their skill at resolving problems improved and visits grew shorter. On average nationally, there was a negligible difference in the number and duration of RN or MSW visits for AIDS patients compared to traditional hospice patients.

It is worth noting that the major part of the national hospice experience thus far has been with gay, white men. There is far less experience to report with the second wave population: IV drug users, women, and children. These are often people of color with far fewer personal resources, financial or human, who enter the treatment system later in the course of the disease. We can assume, therefore, that the financial impact will be generally greater for these patients.

Inpatient Care

Most hospice executives in our survey expected persons with AIDS to have more hospitalizations with longer inpatient stays than traditional hospice patients. In Los Angeles, where two certified hospices provide care in group homes, the hospitalization rate is negligible. Because the staff in these homes are well trained and comfortable with the dying process, hospital admissions for terminal care for these AIDS hospice patients has virtually been eliminated.

The Hospice at Mission Hill in Boston, opened in November, 1989, is an 18-bed inpatient facility for terminally ill AIDS patients with acute care needs. Their daily cost of $320.00 for acute inpatient AIDS care includes $231.00 for personnel and $17.00 for drugs. Initially, medications cost $27.00 per day but when they reexamined the appropriateness of aerosolized pentamidine and AZT, based on patient condition and the purpose of the therapy, they were able to reduce utilization, thus the $10.00 per day reduction in cost.

In Los Angeles Chris Brownlie Hospice, a 25 bed state licensed congregate living health facility considered to be the patient's home, is staffed with LVN's around the clock. The average cost per patient day, excluding prescription drugs, is $200.00. The average length of stay at Brownlie is 37.8 days compared with 23.0 days at Mission Hill.

Private Insurance

Negotiating benefits for patients with AIDS has become a science and an art for hospice programs. Many providers are able to maximize private insurance reimbursement by negotiating modifications in coverage. If a hospice can demonstrate that coordinating care with other agencies such as group homes will prevent hospitalization — thereby reducing overall costs — reimbursers are sometimes flexible in considering and authorizing payment even when there is no specific hospice benefit in the policy. Hospital Home Health Care Agency of California has been successful in persuading insurers to pay the daily room and board rate at the group homes in addition to the cost of hospice services. The only alternative is often an acute care hospital which all would agree is an inappropriate use of human, medical, and financial resources.

Case Management. Individualized case management is an approach employed by many insurance companies to control costs by allowing case managers to determine the most appropriate level of care and cost effective services for patients. Case management as a delivery modality and the AIDS epidemic have developed side by side (Beresford, 1988).

John Hancock Mutual Life Insurance Company has been in the vanguard of exploring new strategies for treating AIDS beneficiaries while at the same time controlling costs. Under Hancock's case management program, a patient can request a case manager who will make coverage exceptions aimed at keeping the patient out of the hospital.

Steven Peskin, Hancock's Medical Director, points out that, "The average cost of AIDS today is $60,000 to $75,000 per patient from diagnosis to death; through case management, Hancock is slicing $30,000 from the bill, primarily by keeping patients out of the hospital" (Mahar, 1989; p. 20).

Despite these few glimmers of light, there is still considerable confusion and ignorance about hospice care within the private insurance industry. Steven Zembo, Vice President for Operations of Health Resources Management in San Francisco, advises clients to put together a complete information dossier on a case before calling the insurance company. Since this initiates a dialogue and provides a starting point for negotiation, he allows the company's claims representatives to then describe benefit coverage before proposing alternatives. Once benefits have been explained, Zembo requests the case management option or, if this is not available, asks to speak to the claims supervisor.

Many hospice providers will negotiate a per diem rate at this point, using the Medicare daily rate as the floor, not the ceiling, for reimbursement. It is advisable for the hospice to determine how frequently the insurance company demands clinical reports. Often, a weekly verbal update reduces the need for written communications. To succeed in maximizing private reimbursement requires persistence, assertiveness, creativity, and consistent follow through (Beresford, 1988).

Unreimbursed Care

That approximately 10%-15% of persons with AIDS cared for by hospices have no medical coverage is a sobering reality. One of the basic tenets of American hospice care has always been that hospices would provide care without consideration of a patient's ability to pay. To meet this challenge, some hospice programs have raised funds in their communities specifically to care for indigent persons with AIDS. In our Fall 1990 survey, directors of hospice programs in several communities where AIDS is not prevalent mentioned their initial hesitation about making public their program's involvement in caring for persons with AIDS. This took on a special irony, in that they were actively seeking funds specifically for AIDS care. In Stamford, Connecticut and Santa Rosa, California the decision to appeal directly to the community was not met with the anticipated backlash, and support has been forthcoming. Other programs remain cautious because the community is so closed-minded about those with HIV disease.

Meeting the Challenge

It is evident, then, that caring for persons with AIDS incorporates a number of challenges, not the least of which is the financial. As the number of diagnosed people continues to rise, and as cities and states become more overwhelmed with the costs of caring for those with HIV infection, the role of hospice in the continuum of care will become more appreciated.

Although the hospice executives in our survey whose agencies have cared for persons with AIDS spoke of various approaches in maximizing existing resources or seeking new funding, most of them acknowledged the need to identify program limits. Some allocated a specific dollar amount for unreimbursed care; others raised funds for attendant care and worked within that limitation. Not one single hospice director responding to our survey indicated an inability to accommodate the needs of terminally ill persons with AIDS.

ORGANIZATIONAL MODELS OF HOSPICE RESPONSE TO THE AIDS EPIDEMIC

This section will highlight the responses of several hospice programs to the HIV epidemic. These programs, through the development of relationships with other HIV service providers in their communities, have brought about realistic yet creative solutions. As part of the process, they have also assumed an assured place in the continuum of care for those with HIV disease.

Residential Hospice Care: A Collaborative Model

In Los Angeles, the gay community's response to the epidemic was the development of several residences or "hospice houses" for those infected with HIV. It became obvious to us at the Hospice of the Hospital Home Health Care Agency of California that it was going to be impossible, given the limited resources of most of these small community-based organizations, for them to continue to provide professional medical and nursing care with volunteers. Our offer to provide the expertise of the hospice team to the residents of one of the AIDS houses was met with welcome relief.

Initially we worked out a formal relationship with one community based organization, then with two others. These arrangements have clarified working relationships between the hospice and the community agencies. The house manager is responsible for the day to day operation of the house, including the attendant care staff, and the hospice is responsible for the professional care. In this way the house manager functions as a primary caregiver, relying on the guidance and advice of the hospice team.

Although it is more complicated to work with another autonomous organization, the benefits are considerable. Scarce resources are shared and the strengths of both organizations are maximized. The hospice is able to bill Medicaid for professional care and the house is able to charge a room and board rate. At City of Angels Hospice House, the average cost per day is $150.00. If a patient has private insurance, that charge will often be covered. Otherwise, a patient will contribute up to $30.00 per day from monthly Supplemental Security Income (SSI) payments. Both organizations, then, share the burden of caring for those patients for whom there is no reimbursement.

Networking

The belief that a comprehensive community model would serve the diverse needs of HIV infected people, led Paul Brenner, when he was with the Hospice of Palm Beach County, to integrate key providers of HIV services in the county into a network of cooperative relationships. His achievement was to develop an array of services that would enable an HIV infected individual to receive appropriate care, irrespective of where he or she entered the system.

Among the several providers were drug treatment programs, legal aid services, the County Health Department, and Catholic Charities, to name a few. The network was so successful that Hospice of Palm Beach was selected as one of nine case management projects funded nationwide in 1986 by the Robert Wood Johnson Foundation. The original consortium of providers has evolved into the Comprehensive AIDS Program of Palm Beach.

Hospice Staff Involvement in the Community

In our survey as we spoke to hospice program directors across the country, a need almost always mentioned was for hospice staff to become actively involved in the HIV service network.

Carolyn Fitzpatrick-Cassin of Hospice of Southeastern Michigan saw a sharp increase in referrals of AIDS patients in 1990 as a result of her participation in a consortium of AIDS health care providers. The cooperation and mutual support among the members has resulted in each provider utilizing each others' programs, thus maximizing services. Again, the total burden of caring for persons with AIDS does not rest solely with the hospice.

That you cannot do this work alone is a lesson that each hospice program learns early. Just as no individual hospice nurse or social worker can provide all the expertise and support needed for any one patient and family, neither can a hospice program meet all the needs of persons with AIDS who are referred to it. If the hospice program knows how to utilize a "Buddy" program for volunteer assistance or a Being Alive support group, those resources can be offered to AIDS patients and families.

By taking a proactive position in the HIV service network, a hospice is visibly playing a vital role. The initial reluctance of AIDS groups to refer to hospice care can be countered as other service providers learn firsthand about the philosophy and approach of individual programs toward AIDS care. Similarly, opportunities for funding increase when several organizations put forth a coordinated effort. AIDS Project Los Angeles (APLA), the largest AIDS service organization in Southern California, as a response to the increased demand for services and their great success in fund raising, made an unprecedented contribution of $225,000 to 11 community based organizations whose services benefit APLA clients.

Across the country hospice programs are joining with other HIV service providers in sponsoring AIDS Walkathons, Marathons, and other fundraising events. This approach is especially effective in communities that can support a number of deserving organizations with one event. Early in the epidemic, specialized programs for caring for persons with AIDS were developed out of necessity. In the years to come, however, "Growth in the numbers of persons needing care will make it impossible in many areas to maintain separate and specialized programs. HIV-infected persons will ultimately have to become integrated within the health care delivery system as a whole" (Morrison, 1990; p. 3).

AIDS Case Management

In 1985 the California State Legislature, eager to spread the means of success of San Francisco in containing the costs of AIDS care to other areas, began a state-wide demonstration of case management and home care services. In 1987 the State Office of AIDS began funding projects in communities outside the major metropolitan areas that had a much lower incidence of AIDS.

The Board of Directors of Hospice Caring Project of Santa Cruz County voted to expand their services to AIDS patients and applied for, and were awarded state funding to carry out the case management model in the county. Despite the relatively few diagnosed AIDS patients, 93 in 1989, that number represented a doubling since 1987 (Littman & Siemsen, 1989).

Like many communities outside major metropolitan areas, Santa Cruz County has limited public and community health care services. Patients with AIDS must rely on private hospitals, individual medical practitioners, and private social and health services agencies. The numbers of AIDS patients are insufficient to support specialized programs anywhere in the system.

The case management model that worked well in large metropolitan areas where there is an existing system of coordination among inpatient, outpatient, and community-based services, has been adapted to fit the smaller Santa Cruz County. JoAnn Siemsen of the Hospice Caring Project reports that because of their expanded role in the community, hospice care is now more readily accepted. Indeed, the hospice has cared for more than 50% of all patients who have died in Santa Cruz. Siemsen notes, "The fact that we are not taking the risk alone has enabled us to continue to reaffirm our commitment and to seek solutions to decreased funding and increased needs" (J. Siemsen, personal communication, September 27, 1990). A waiting list has been instituted so that scarce resources can now be allocated in an equitable manner. The Health Services Agency of Santa Cruz County has also created a drug fund to cover the cost of medications not otherwise reimbursed.

In Miami, Hospice, Inc. has developed a separate service for persons with AIDS called Project Outreach which provides services for persons with AIDS who are not appropriate for either hospice or for high-tech home care services. This pilot project, funded through several sources, represents another form of expansion of services by an experienced hospice provider.

Clearly, not every hospice program is willing or able to make the decision to expand services in these ways. The most important step for any hospice considering it is to examine its commitment to caring for persons with AIDS and its ability to do so.

CONCLUSION

Although the data about the costs of caring for terminally ill persons with AIDS are, at this time, very limited, it is fair to say that those patients utilize more resources than traditional hospice patients. Among experienced providers there is agreement that persons with AIDS at some time may require longer and more frequent nursing and social work visits, more attendant level care, more supplies, more numerous and more expensive medications; and that their emotional, psychological, spiritual, and financial needs can be overwhelming.

There is also agreement, on the other hand, that hospices have a moral and ethical obligation to extend their services, to the degree feasible and fitting, to care for persons with AIDS. The extension of services may necessitate changes in admission criteria and/or the development of new relationships with other HIV service providers. Hospices may decide to allocate a percentage of fundraising dollars to persons with AIDS or they may contribute to the development of residential day care programs for them.

In order to respond in a fiscally responsible way, each hospice must revisit its mission and purpose, consider its resources, and make a clear decision about the role it chooses to play in the epidemic in its community. Boston AIDS activist Paul Wright adds that hospices need to be flexible with AIDS patients, but, ". . . not apologetic about what hospice is, where it comes from, what it seeks to offer. I think it's important to think of hospice as an invitation to the patient. It is an opportunity to consider alternatives and to collaborate in his or her own life's journey, even if that journey is close to the end. Hospice offers an opportunity to demonstrate what it means to celebrate life in a very different way—an opportunity for people to reflect and to gather bits and pieces of their lives" (Beresford, 1989; p. 10).

REFERENCES

Beresford, L. (1988, Fall). Private insurance reimbursement. *California Hospice Report, 6*(4), 1-12.

Beresford, L. (1989, Summer/Fall). The challenge of AIDS. *California Hospice Report, 1*(3), 1-16.

CDC (September 1990) U.S. Department of Health and Human Services, *HIV/ AIDS Surveillance*.

Green, J., & Arno, P.S. (1990). The Medicaidization of AIDS. *Journal of the American Medical Association. 264*, 1261-1266.

Littman, E., & Siemsen, J. (1989). AIDS case management. *Caring, 8*(11), 79-84.

Mahar, M. (1989, March 13). Pitiless scourge separating out the hype from hope on AIDS. *Barron's, 7*, 16, 20.

Morrison, C. (1990). Guest editor's perspective. *Pride Institute Journal of Long Term Health Care, 9*, 3.

National Hospice Organization. (1988). *National Hospice Organization Census*.

National Hospice Organization. (1989). *National Hospice Organization Census*.

A Comparison of the Psychosocial Needs of Hospice Patients with AIDS and Those with Other Diagnoses

Nancy Tish Baker
Robert D. Seager

SUMMARY. We compared the amount of psychosocial support required and received by patients with AIDS and without AIDS at Cedar Valley Hospice, Waterloo, Iowa. Hospice patients with AIDS (N = 11) required significantly more psychosocial support than non-AIDS patients (N = 36) of the same average age. The amount of non-hospice social support — family, congregation, and neighbors — received by AIDS patients was significantly less than that received by those with other diagnoses due to a virtual lack of neighbor support. There were no significant differences in family or congregational support. The high level of family support and lack of neighbor support may have been a result of many (8) of the AIDS patients having moved back to the area to die. A survey of hospice staff showed they felt working with AIDS patients was both more time consuming and more stressful than working with patients with other diagnoses.

Nancy Tish Baker, MA in Counseling, is Bereavement Counselor with Cedar Valley Hospice, Waterloo, IA. Robert D. Seager, PhD in Genetics, is Associate Professor of Biology, University of Northern Iowa, Cedar Falls, IA; scientific advisor to the AIDS Coalition of Northeast Iowa; and a member of the board and treasurer of the Cedar Valley AIDS Crisis Fund.

The authors thank Cheryl Hoerner, Executive Director of Cedar Valley Hospice, Kathleen Muleady Seager, and Robert Lembke for their support, and Mary Howard for statistical help.

Address correspondence to Robert D. Seager, Department of Biology, University of Northern Iowa, McCollum Science Hall 2438, Cedar Falls, IA 50614.

INTRODUCTION

The argument has been made that the psychosocial needs of persons with AIDS should be no different than those of people terminally ill with other diseases. Like AIDS, many cancers, degenerative neurological conditions, and Alzheimer's Disease to name a few are dreaded and do not respond well to treatment. But AIDS is truly different. Since it is most often acquired through drug use and homosexual activity, it carries a profound stigma (Nichols & Ostrow, 1984). People with AIDS tend to be young and the young do not expect to die (Tiblier et al., 1989). Changes in body image, self-esteem, daily habits, sense of control, and general lifestyle can be rapid and precipitous in people with AIDS. These changes are usually more dramatic than in people with other potentially terminal diseases in whom decline may be more gradual (Nichols & Ostrow, 1984).

Forstein (1984) contended that the psychosocial impact of AIDS on a person could only be understood by equating it with the problems of minorities in our society. Persons with AIDS must endure social reactions that affect their self-esteem and foster feelings of alienation and isolation.

Since many persons with AIDS are already ostracized by society, they do not have the family, congregation, and community ties that usually provide psychosocial support to a dying person (Nichols & Ostrow, 1988). Persons with AIDS have fewer resources available to them, and the health care and psychosocial professionals assisting them are often not trained to deal with their specific problems.

A key issue new to psychotherapists is that for many persons with AIDS, the diagnosis forces an intense crisis. Clients must reveal a lifestyle that is possibly unacceptable to their families of origin at the same time as they are disclosing their diagnosis of a potentially fatal illness (Tiblier et al., 1989). The level of stress is elevated even further if the person with AIDS has conflicts of loyalty between the family of origin and lovers, or other significant others.

THE STUDY

In this study, we compared the amount of psychosocial support required by and given to hospice patients with AIDS with that given to non-AIDS hospice patients of the same average age. We also measured the amount of social support that each group received from family, congregation, and neighbors. In addition, we surveyed hospice staff members who cared for AIDS patients about their perceptions of the similarities and differences between working with AIDS and with non-AIDS patients.

MATERIALS AND METHODS

Data on age, gender, diagnosis, number of days enrolled in hospice, number of telephone and direct (in person) contacts made by the psychosocial staff, and quality of the non-hospice support system were obtained from the charts of hospice patients who had died or left the Cedar Valley Hospice, Waterloo, Iowa between 1985 and 1990. A total of 12 AIDS patients was identified. One elderly female AIDS patient was excluded from the study due to age. The sample consisted of 11 AIDS patients and 36 non-AIDS patients, all fifty years old or younger. All of the AIDS patients in the sample were male as were 22 (61%) of the non-AIDS patients. The non-hospice support system was subdivided into family, congregation, and neighbors. A support scale of 0 (no support) to 5 (excellent support) was assigned to each subdivision providing a range of 0 to 15 for overall support system. The number of telephone and direct psychosocial staff contacts per patient was divided by the number of days in hospice care and multiplied by 7 to give the average number of contacts per week.

Comparisons between AIDS and non-AIDS patients were done by t-test when variances were homogeneous and by approximate t-test when variances were heterogeneous (Sokal & Rohlf, 1989.) Variance homogeneity was determined by F-test (Sokal & Rohlf, 1969.)

A seven item questionnaire probing staff perceptions about the time and stress associated with working with AIDS versus non-AIDS patients was administered to the nurses, psychosocial team members and other staff (N = 13) of Cedar Valley Hospice who worked with AIDS patients. We asked (1) whether AIDS patients *required* more time than similarly aged patients without AIDS, and if so, (2) how much more time, (3) whether more time was *given* to AIDS patients, (4) if so, why, (5) whether younger patients in general required more time, (6) whether it was more stressful to work with AIDS patients than non-AIDS patients of similar age, and (7) if so, why working with AIDS patients was more stressful. Some questions were not answered by some respondents.

RESULTS

There was no significant difference between the AIDS and non-AIDS patients in average age. Although the AIDS patients were enrolled in hospice one and one-half times longer, this difference was not statistically significant (Table 1). There was, however, a significant difference in the total number of psychosocial staff contacts made to AIDS patients per week ($p = < .026$) (see Table 1). AIDS patients required contact over 2 1/2 times as often by telephone and over twice as often in person (see Figure 1). There was also a significant difference in the amount of family/community support received ($p = < .024$) (see Table 1), due primarily to the virtual lack of a neighbor support for AIDS patients (see Figure 2).

The perceptions of the hospice staff agreed with these results. Ninety-two percent felt that patients with AIDS always or usually required and were given more time than patients of similar age without AIDS. The nursing staff estimated spending fifteen minutes to an hour more per visit with these patients.

Most respondents (92%) felt that extra time was needed because AIDS patients had more physical and more emotional needs. Specific reasons for giving extra time included staying to talk "beyond the nurse stuff" because AIDS patients, ". . . not only had more physical demands, due to the roller coaster nature of the disease, but were unsupported by the general community and emotionally devastated," that ". . . because every case is so different with so many complications that are so unpredictable, fear of the unknown is always more frightening for these patients," and there was ". . . less support and more unresolved issues and conflicts with gay and/or drug issues."

Although most respondents (74%) felt that younger patients in general required more time, the majority (64%) also felt that working with AIDS patients was more stressful than working with non-AIDS patients of similar ages. Reasons included their unique needs and their social stigmatization.

Table 1. A comparison of age, days enrolled in hospice, hospice staff
contacts, and non-hospice social support for hospice patients with AIDS
and with other diagnoses.

STUDY VARIABLES	HOSPICE PATIENTS WITH AIDS (N=11)		HOSPICE PATIENTS WITH OTHER DIAGNOSES (N=36)		
	MEAN	STANDARD ERROR	MEAN	STANDARD ERROR	p
Age	31.5	1.6	34.4	2.4	0.337
Days enrolled in hospice	150.1	35.8	93.3	20.3	0.180
Total hospice staff contacts/week	2.8	0.6	1.2	0.2	0.026*
Non-hospice social support score	7.4	1.1	10.6	0.7	0.024*

* p<0.05

65

FIGURE 1. PSYCHOSOCIAL CONTACTS MADE BY HOSPICE STAFF

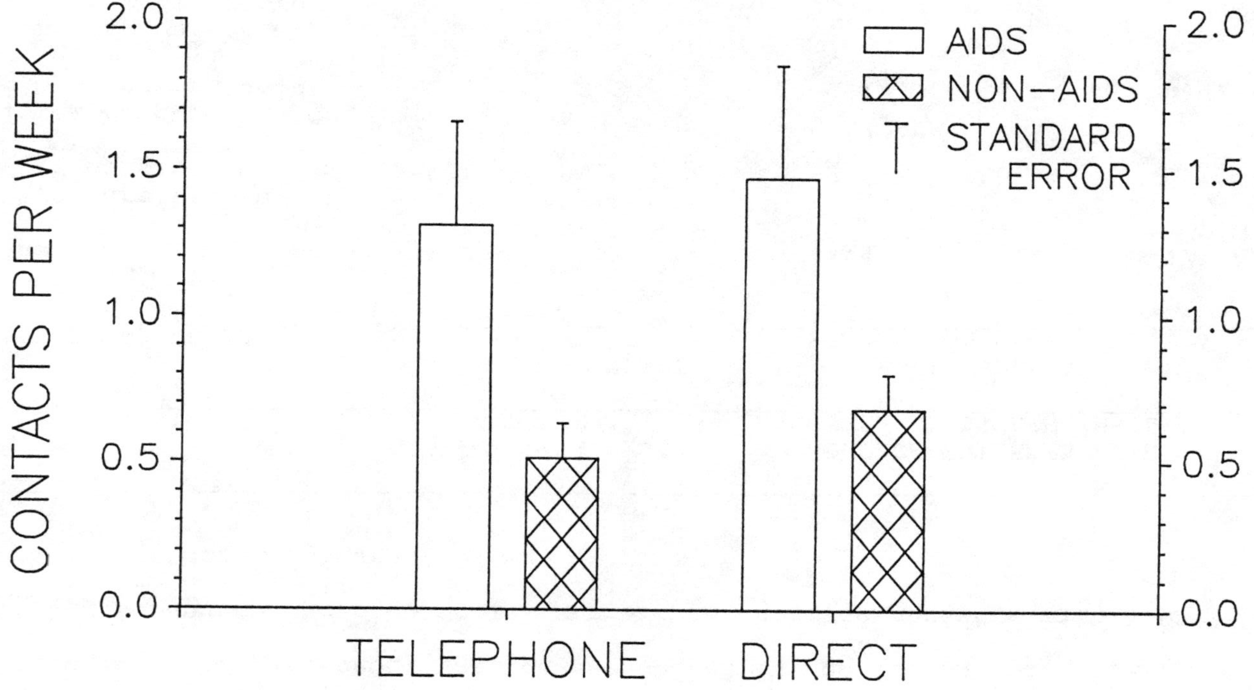

AIDS
NON-AIDS
STANDARD ERROR

CONTACTS PER WEEK

TELEPHONE   DIRECT

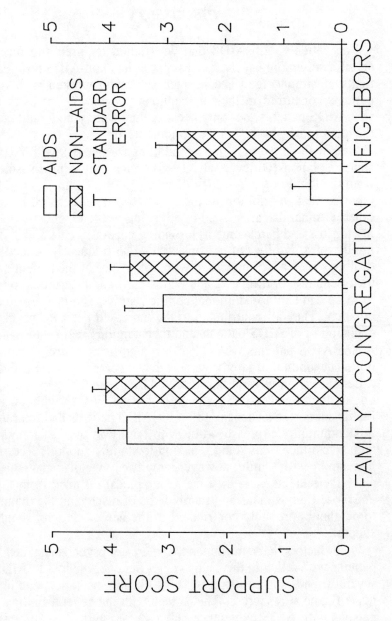

FIGURE 2. NON-HOSPICE SOCIAL SUPPORT

67

DISCUSSION

The patients with AIDS that we studied required and received significantly more psychosocial support than non-AIDS hospice patients of similar age. The hospice staff who worked with AIDS patients concurred in their perceptions that they spent extra time with AIDS patients, not only because they were young but because they had more physical and emotional needs.

One of the most egregious conditions for persons with AIDS is social isolation (Dilley et al., 1985), often extending to isolation from the family of origin (Schofferman 1988). Tiblier et al. (1989) reported that in addition to the psychosocial burdens common to other terminal diseases, such as adjusting to the diagnosis, preparing for loss and bereavement, providing necessary care and shifting family roles, families of persons with AIDS frequently needed help dealing with fears of infection, with acceptance of the patient's sexual orientation or drug use, and with stigma and discrimination. All of these can lead to additional conflict, stress, and need for reconciliation. They all contributed to the increased need for psychosocial support of AIDS patients and their families in this study.

The AIDS patients we studied had significantly less social support. The amount of family support they received, however, did not differ significantly from that received by non-AIDS patients. Only one of the eleven AIDS patients in our study was without some family support. Since many (8) of the AIDS patients had returned to this community expressly to be with family in the last months of their lives, there was some selection for family support. Returning home to be with family, however, amplified overall social isolation since the patients were at some geographical distance from lovers and close friends. This and family fears of disclosing the diagnosis to neighbors probably contributed to the general lack of neighbor support.

Other factors that contributed to the greater psychosocial needs of patients with AIDS in this study were grief over the loss to AIDS of several friends and co-workers, lack of health insurance, and inadequate financial resources. This agreed with the general finding that persons with AIDS experience helplessness, guilt, loss of control, denial, anger, depression, anxiety, bereavement due to multiple losses, legal, financial, social and medical problems, loss of income, and unemployment and housing concerns (Nichols & Ostrow, 1984). Many of the patients with AIDS had been bright, active, and productive people. All of them lost control of nearly every aspect of their lives.

Meeting the complex needs of a patient with AIDS, ". . . is an unprecedented challenge for those providing home hospice care" (Martin 1988, p. 465) and serving patients with AIDS requires significantly more time and causes more stress to staff. The results of this study strongly support Schofferman (1988, p. 445) who stated that, ". . . psychosocial issues are so complex that they often dominate the clinical picture of the person dying of AIDS."

REFERENCES

Dilley, J.W., Ochitill, H.N., Perl, M., & Volberding, P.A. (1985). Findings in psychiatric consultations with patients with acquired immune deficiency syndrome. *American Journal of Psychiatry, 142*(1), 82-86.

Forstein, M. (1984). The psychosocial impact of the acquired immunodeficiency syndrome, *Seminars in Oncology, 11*(1), 77-82.

Martin, J.P. (1988). Hospice and home care for persons with AIDS/ARC: Meeting the challenges and ensuring quality. *Death Studies, 12*(5-6) 463-480.

Nichols, S.E., & Ostrow, D.G. (1984). *Psychiatric Implications of Acquired Immune Deficiency Syndrome.* American Psychiatric Press, Inc., Washington, D.C.

Schofferman, J. (1988). Care of the AIDS patient. *Death Studies, 12*(5-6) 433-449.

Sokal, R.R. & Rohlf, R.J. (1969). *Biometry.* San Francisco: W.H. Freeman and Company.

Tiblier, K.B., Walker, G., & Rolland, J.S. (1989). Therapeutic issues when working with families of persons with AIDS. *AIDS and Families.* New York: The Haworth Press, Inc.

Family Adaptation to AIDS:
A Comparative Study

Ronnie Atkins
Madalon O'Rawe Amenta

SUMMARY. In this study the McCubbin stress and coping model was used as a theoretical framework to compare the differences in family adaptation to AIDS and to other terminal illnesses. The non-probability convenience sample consisted of 26 families of AIDS patients and 26 of hospice patients with other terminal illnesses. The Family Inventory of Life Events and Changes was used to measure the number of stressful events experienced by the family since diagnosis and the Family Adaptation to Medical Stressors Questionnaire measured role flexibility. Families of AIDS patients had significantly more stress, more rules prohibiting emotional expression, lower trust levels, and more illness anxiety than the other families.

INTRODUCTION

The feelings endured to some extent by most dying people and their families — fear, guilt, helplessness, depression, anger, confusion, despair — are experienced by persons with AIDS and their families even more intensely. In addition, persons with AIDS and their families feel marked social stigma, fear of contagion, fear of infection, fear of abandonment, and economic hardship (Christ & Weiner, 1985; Helquist, 1987; Macklin, 1988; Giaquinta, 1989). There have been many studies about individuals with an AIDS diag-

Ronnie Atkins, RN, MSN, is Assistant Director and Director of Nursing at Saint Anthony's Hospital Hospice and Life Enrichment Center, Amarillo, TX. Madalon O'Rawe Amenta, RN, DPH, is Associate Professor of Nursing, at The Pennsylvania State University, McKeesport Campus, McKeesport, PA.

Address correspondence to Ronnie Atkins, 2113 South Hayden Street, Amarillo, TX 79109.

nosis and the impact the progress of the disease has had on their lives and the lives of their families. To our knowledge, however, there have been no reported studies relating family adaptation to an AIDS diagnosis using a family systems theoretical model. In this study we compared the adaptation of clients with AIDS and their families to that of hospice clients terminally ill with other diseases and their families using the McCubbin and Patterson Double ABCX model (1983).

THE MODEL

Systems theory posits that a stress or burden on one element of the system will affect all the other parts. Role theory maintains that when one member of a system such as the family becomes chronically ill, his or her responsibilities and tasks must be assumed by others. This will, perforce, cause stress until a new level of balance in family functioning is achieved.

All stress within a system, however, does not necessarily lead to crisis. Crisis results when the stresses exceed the person's or the system's ability to manage through reliance on habitual problem-solving strategies to achieve equilibrium. When tension mounts beyond this point the person or the system calls on habitual emergency problem solving measures. If these do not produce relief and the stresses still remain threatening to integrity, the person or the system enters a stage of confusion or disorganization that is called crisis – a reaction to perceived loss, the threat of loss, or overwhelming challenge (Graves, 1984). In some cases the reaction to the crisis – intense anxiety – becomes internalized and creates an additional inner stress that adds to the total burden. In this self-feeding cyclical system, the potential of risk to the health and well being of the person or group undergoing the crisis becomes great (Detheredge & Johnson, 1986).

Hill (1949; 1958) was one of the first to develop a family crisis model for use in research (see Figure 1). This model focuses on the pre-crisis variables that account for differences in family vulnerability to stress inducing events and hence the onset and the degree of crisis for the family. In this model "A" (the stressful event) interacting with "B" (the family's coping resources) interacting with

FIGURE 1

Diagram of ABCX and Double ABCX Models

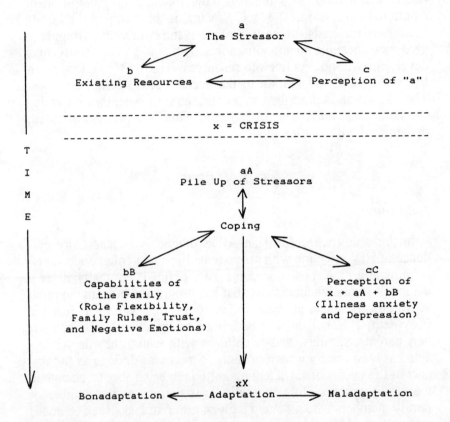

"C" (the meaning the family ascribes to the event) produces "X" (the crisis). This is a descriptive, static, relatively simple formulation.

The Double ABCX model developed by McCubbin and Patterson (1983) adapted Hill's design and focused on the family's adaptation to the crisis by including post-crisis variables and outcomes. In this model the "aA" factor is the pile up of stressful circumstances, or the accumulation of them over time. The "bB" factor arrays the family's capabilities of meeting the demands of the various stressful factors. Among the more important are the family's internal adaptive capacities, the assorted members' personal resources, and the family's social support. This includes role flexibility within the family and family rules regarding the freedom or prohibition of emotional expression. The "cC" factor, is the meaning the family ascribes to the crisis. In the face of crisis the family may struggle to give new meaning to the situation. In this stage the family may develop new, and redefine old resources. The "xX" factor identifies the family's adaptation to the accumulated stresses or crisis. The adaptation is described as a continuum of outcomes reflecting the family's achievement of balance. This is a process oriented, dynamic, more complex model.

THE STUDY

Definitions

In this study we defined an AIDS diagnosis as laboratory evidence of HIV infection with at least one life-threatening opportunistic infection or Kaposi's sarcoma. We defined terminally ill as a diagnosis of malignant disease that has progressed beyond the point at which care aimed at remission or tumor regression was feasible (Cassileth, 1982). Family was defined as the client's spouse/partner, parents, siblings, and/or children with whom the client interacted at least once a month or more. Stress was defined as the impact of life events of sufficient magnitude to bring about a change in the family system. Role flexibility was defined as the number of family members who assumed a given group of tasks such as house cleaning, cooking, caretaking, yard maintenance, marketing or bill paying. Adaptation was defined as the family's capacity to meet obstacles and shift course as a cohesive unit. Social network was defined as the number of people the family felt they could rely on.

The Setting

Data for this study were obtained from clients of a hospice and from those of an AIDS support organization located in a small metropolitan area of approximately 150,000 people. Each agency serves both the metropolitan community and the surrounding rural area of the Texas Panhandle — largely small family farm and ranch country.

The hospice, a 20 bed inpatient facility with a home care division, maintains an average census of 32. The AIDS support organization serves an average of 40 clients. At the time of data collection 44 persons with AIDS had been diagnosed in the Texas Panhandle. This figure does not reflect the many AIDS clients who had returned home to die with their families of origin in the region. Both agencies, despite the diversities in the type of service provided, adhere to the same philosophy. That is to provide supportive care to meet the special needs arising from the physical, emotional, spiritual, and social stresses experienced by dying people and their families.

METHODS

The Sample

The sample was a nonprobability convenience selection of 26 hospice clients and their families and 26 clients and their families from the AIDS support organization. The prospective subjects were selected by the administrators of each agency. Those who did not consent, who were imminently dying, or who could not respond easily and coherently for other reasons were excluded from the study.

The Instruments

Two instruments were used. The Family Inventory of Life Events and Changes (FILE) Scale (McCubbin, Wilson, & Patterson, 1979) measured the number of stress producing factors perceived by the family since the client's diagnosis. This scale of 71 YES/NO items assesses the normative and non-normative life events of the family. A total score is determined by summing the YES responses. The instrument measures nine life change areas derived through factor analysis: intra-family, marital, childbearing, financial, work-family, family care, losses, transition, and legal concerns. The various sections of the scale include from 4 to 17 items. Overall internal reliability is reported as .72 (McCubbin & Patterson, 1981).

The authors report reliability for the FILE scale in terms of

Chronbach's coefficient alpha. The overall scale reliability is 0.81, with subscales varying from 0.73 to 0.30. Validity was determined by discriminant analysis between low conflict and high conflict families (p < .01) (McCubbin, Patterson, & Wilson, 1982).

The second instrument, the Family Adaptation to Medical Stressors (FAMS) scale (Koch, 1983), was used to measure negative emotions, illness anxiety, depression, trust, rules prohibiting emotional expression, and role flexibility. In the development of the scale these dimensions were identified through factor analysis. Each section of this 36 item questionnaire contains 4-8 YES/NO choices with the YES items carrying a value of one, the NO zero. The scoring range for each section varies with the number of items. Chronbach's alpha was 0.75 (Koch, 1983).

Data for the demographic and other descriptive variables were derived from another set of investigator designed questions. These included items about age, income, occupation, employment status at time of interview, education, months since diagnosis, number of people in the social network, and self-rated stress level.

Data Collection and Analysis

One of the authors who worked as a nurse for the hospice and was on the Board of Directors of the AIDS support organization administered the instruments to clients and families during home visits. This was possibly the only route through which the 26 AIDS clients and their families could have come to be known and contacted. The clients and their families both participated in responding to the questionnaires.

After the questionnaires were scored and coded, the data were evaluated for statistical significance using a two-tailed t-test for independent samples. To assure confidentiality, only the researchers had access to the data.

RESULTS

Characteristics of the Sample

Demographic and other selected characteristics of the patients and families in the samples are arrayed in Tables 1 and 2. The persons with AIDS were slightly better educated (14.9 years) com-

Table 1

Gender, Employment Status, and Self-Reported Stress Level of Hospice
and AIDS Support Organization Clients/Families

	Hospice Clients N = 26		AIDS Clients N = 26	
Characteristic	N	Percent	N	Percent
Gender				
Male	11	42.3	26	100.0
Female	15	57.7	-	-
Employment Status				
Full Time	6	23.1	18	69.2
Part Time	5	19.2	2	7.7
Unemployed	15	57.7	6	23.1
Stress Level				
(Self Reported)				
Low	-	-	2	7.7
Medium	14	53.9	10	38.5
High	7	26.9	11	42.3
Very High	5	19.2	3	11.5

pared to the hospice patients (12.8). The persons with AIDS (mean
age 35) were a generation younger than the hospice patients (mean
age 59). Although, each group had slightly less average annual income both at the time of the interviews (persons with AIDS
$22,000, hospice patients $25,000) than prior to illness (persons
with AIDS $24,000, hospice patients $28,000), the spread in income in both groups differed. Both prior to and at time of interview
the persons with AIDS showed far more variation around the mean.

The profiles of the two groups' employment status at the time of
the interviews demonstrated an almost perfect isometric inversion.

Table 2

Age, Income, Education, Time Since Diagnosis, and Size of Social Network
in Hospice and AIDS Support Organization Clients/Families

Characteristic	Hospice Clients N = 26		AIDS Clients N = 26	
	Mean	SD	Mean	SD
Age	59	19.8	35	6.9 *
Annual Family Income				
Current	25,000	22,000	22,000	13,000
Prior to Illness	28,000	21,000	24,000	9,000
Years of Education of Client	12.8	2.7	14.9	2.5
Months Since Diagnosis	13.5	10.1	19.0	10.7
Number in Family Social Network	10.2	7.1	6.2	5.6 *

* $p < .05$

Twenty-three percent of the hospice patients were employed full
time; 23% of the persons with AIDS were unemployed. Con-
versely, 69% of the persons with AIDS were employed full time;
58% of the hospice patients were unemployed. On average the persons with AIDS had lived longer since diagnosis (19 months) than
the hospice patients (13.5 months). The persons with AIDS on av-

erage also had statistically significantly fewer numbers of people in their social networks (6.2) than the hospice patients (10.2) (p < .05). The two groups did not differ on self-reported levels of stress. Fifty-six and one tenth percent of the hospice patients/families and 53.8 % of the persons with AIDS and families reported high to very high stress.

FILE and FAMS Scores

The mean differences in the scores for accumulated stresses measured by the FILE scale for persons with AIDS and their families, 20.54; and for the hospice patients and their families, 15.19 were statistically significant (p < .05) (see Table 3). On the FAMS questionnaire, there were no statistically significant differences between the scores of the two groups on role flexibility, depression, or negative emotions. The two groups did, however, differ statistically significantly on the trust, anxiety, and rules prohibiting emotional expression dimensions. The persons with AIDS and their families registered less trust, more rules prohibiting emotional expression, and more illness anxiety than did the hospice patients and their families.

DISCUSSION

The persons with AIDS/families' documentation of significantly greater pile-up of stresses is not surprising. There are several reasons why this might be so. AIDS is an especially devastating disease. It is infectious, fatal, there is currently no cure, and although many persons with AIDS do not, they can live three years or more after diagnosis. This extended time that a person and family must live under the threat of imminent death keeps a crisis state alive. Persons with AIDS have been infectious for many years prior to the onset of symptoms and they remain infected and infectious for life (Legislative Task Force on AIDS, 1988). The disease strikes young adults whom we customarily think of as having their best and brightest years still ahead of them. These young adults, especially the homosexuals, are frequently at the beginning of, or in the mid-

Table 3

FILE and FAMS Results for Families of AIDS Clients and Those of
Hospice Clients Terminally Ill With Other Diagnoses

Scale	Range	AIDS (26)		Hospice (26)		t- value
		M	SD	M	SD	
FILE (pile up	0-71	20.54	8.05	15.19	10.39	-2.07 *
of stressors)						
FAMS						
Role Flexibility	0-6	1.77	1.34	1.88	0.99	0.35
Rules Prohibiting	0-4	3.24	0.90	2.73	1.56	-1.96 *
Emotional Expression						
Trust	0-5	1.58	0.95	2.15	0.97	2.18 *
Illness Anxiety	0-6	4.50	1.07	3.24	1.86	-2.56 *
Depression	0-4	3.58	1.53	3.19	1.36	-0.96
Negative Emotions	0-4	3.77	1.88	4.23	1.48	0.98

*p < .05

dle of very promising careers. They have productive and creative
human potential in which our society places high value.

Because they are young, they often do not have the financial
resources to call on that older people with a hospice care eligible
illness might have. Although the persons with AIDS/families in this
study did not have markedly lower income at time of interview,
neither did they have the medical insurance benefits that older people, eligible for Medicare would have. It had been on average 19
months since diagnosis for the persons with AIDS/families, so
many of them may have had more than 5 months to go before quali-
fying for SSI benefits. The cost of the disease is potentially far more

ruinous to persons with AIDS/families than the costs of hospice care for a malignancy to older patients' families.

Since AIDS first occurred in stigmatized groups, homosexual men and intravenous drug abusers, the social reaction to those with the disease has been confounded by moralistic assignments of "blaming the victims" (National Academy of Science, 1988; Sontag, 1988). This enhances the anxiety many people tend to feel when they must confront fatal and infectious diseases. These are all increased burdens that persons with AIDS/families are subject to and which can be internalized into the self-feeding cycle that keeps a crisis viable.

The finding that the persons with AIDS and their families had statistically significantly more rules prohibiting emotional expression, less trust, and more illness anxiety may have been a result of the social and physiological factors stated above. It also may have contributed to an accumulation in intensity of the stresses.

The lack of statistical significance in role flexibility between the two groups, and their very close scores at the low end of the scale, might reflect the norm of the rural community from which both groups came. The ethos of the rural community might also account for the similarities in scores between the two groups on self reported levels of stress in contrast to the statistically significant differences in the FILE scores. Just as role flexibility is not a widely found characteristic of rural families, who tend to be more traditionally rigid in role assignment, so not acknowledging stress (read: not telling everybody your troubles) may be customary, as well.

These families are used to containing their stress. They cannot/ will not talk openly about life style or sexual habits. Dying is perhaps just one more stressful event that they accept and deal with stoically as they do the other major factors in their lives that are routinely kept secret.

That the PWA/families had significantly fewer people in their social networks also points up a more stressful condition that these people must endure. It is likely that there are fewer people in persons with AIDS/families' social networks due to the stigma attached to the disease and the fears emanating from its infectiousness. This lower number of people close enough to be able to help in practical ways and to give emotional and social support would also contribute to an increase in stress levels. One of the greatest fears of the dying, no matter what the disease or terminal condition, is the fear of abandonment.

IMPLICATIONS FOR FURTHER RESEARCH AND PRACTICE

The results of this study provide additional statistical underpinnings for many of the intuitive assumptions that have been made about the differences between persons with AIDS/families and patients/families with traditional hospice diagnoses. With this knowledge hospice programs ought better be able to devise modifications of the traditional hospice model to suit the diverse needs of families of persons with AIDS. Hospice workers can develop increased sensitivity to the characteristic stresses and added total stress burden these families bear. Hospice programs might also contribute to an increase in numbers in the support network for these families by encouraging staff to volunteer as "buddies." With their training and experience and the support techniques they have developed for traditional hospice care, they can help elicit therapeutic emotional expression in a safe environment, help increase levels of trust through acceptance, and allay illness anxiety of persons with AIDS.

The Double ABCX model might serve as the basis of a patient/family assessment protocol for all patient groups and their families. With the model in mind, clinicians can be anticipating reactions and behaviors as they note the elements accumulating at the apices of the triangle. They can elicit families' definition of the event as a powerful working tool in helping families structure adaptation. Finally, in a well-designed protocol, the xX dimension would help in identifying helpful processes and delineating progress toward and actual outcomes *vis à vis* adaptation.

Further studies comparing urban and rural groups of AIDS patients and their families should find insights in these data and in the discussion section of the paper. The results of further studies should aid in providing the framework for the development of AIDS support and hospice programs in rural areas.

REFERENCES

Cassileth, P. A. (1982). Common medical complications. In E. R. Cassileth & P. A. Cassileth (Eds.), *Clinical Care of the Terminal Cancer Patient*. Philadelphia: Tea & Febiger.

Christ, G. H., & Wiener, L. S. (1985). Psychological issues in AIDS. In V. DeVita, S. Hellman, & S. Rosenberg (Eds.), *AIDS: Etiology diagnosis, treatment, and prevention*. (pp. 275-279). New York: J. B. Lippincott.

Detherage, K., & Johnson, S. (1986). Primary prevention in stress and crisis. In Edelman, C. & C. Mandle (Eds.) *Health Promotion Throughout the Lifespan*. (pp. 159-181). St. Louis: C.V. Mosby.

Giacquinta, B. (1989). Researching the effects of AIDS on families. *The American Journal of Hospice Care 6* (3), 31-36.

Graves, P. (1984). Intervening in crisis. In Stanhope, M. & J. Lancaster (Eds). *Community Health Nursing: Process and Practice for Promoting Health*. (pp. 405-432). St. Louis: C. V. Mosby.

Helquist, M. (1987). From the heart: The family's response. In B. Moffatt, J. Spiegel, S. Parrish, & M. Helquist (Eds.), *AIDS: A self-care manual* (pp. 26-29). Los Angeles: AIDS Project.

Hill, R. (1949). *Families under Stress*. New York: Harper & Brothers.

Hill, R. (1958). Genetic features of families under stress. *Social Casework, 49*, 139-150.

Koch, A. (1983). Family Adaptation to medical stressors. *Family Systems Medicine, 1*, 78-87.

Legislative Task Force on AIDS (1988). *Statement on preliminary findings*. August, TX: Author.

Macklin, E. (1988). AIDS: Implications for families. *Family Relations, 37*, 141-149.

McCubbin, H. I., & Patterson, J. M. (1983). The family stress process: the double ABCX model of adjustment and adaptation. In H. McCubbin, M. Sussman, & J. Patterson (Eds.), *Social Stress and the family: Advances and developments in family stress theory and research* (pp. 7-39). New York: The Haworth Press, Inc.

McCubbin, H.I., Patterson, J.M., & Wilson, M. (1982). Family inventory of life events and changes. In D.H. Olson, H.I. McCubbin, H. Barnes et al. (Eds.), *Family inventories* (p. 69). St. Paul, MN: Family Social Science, University of Minnesota.

McCubbin, H. I., Wilson, L., & Patterson, J. M. (1979). *Family inventory of life events and changes*. Forbe, MN: University of Minnesota.

National Academy of Sciences (1988). *Confronting AIDS*. Washington, DC: National Academy Press.

Sontag, S. *AIDS and its Metaphors*. (1988). New York: Farrar, Straus and Giroux.

Volunteers Under Threat: AIDS Hospice Volunteers Compared to Volunteers in a Traditional Hospice

I. Michael Shuff
Arthur M. Horne
Nancy G. Westberg
Scott P. Mooney
C.W. Mitchell

SUMMARY. We studied volunteers in one of the world's first AIDS-dedicated hospices and compared them on demographic, experiential, and personality related dimensions to volunteers in a traditional hospice. Eighty percent of the active volunteers at each facility participated. Eight of 16 demographic and 4 of 11 personality related variables differentiated the two groups. AIDS hospice volunteers were on all measures a more heterogeneous group — largely gay or bisexual, younger, more likely to have had prior personal experience with AIDS. In addition, they perceived themselves to be functioning under a significantly higher degree of threat caused by their volunteer work. We performed a post hoc analysis controlling for sexual orientation and matching heterosexual volunteers for gender. Threats to health, social world, employment, and total threat significantly differentiated the two heterosexual groups of volunteers.

I. Michael Shuff, PhD, is Assistant Professor, Department of Counseling, Indiana State University; Arthur M. Horne, PhD, is Chairman and Director of the Department of Training in Counseling Psychology at the University of Georgia. Nancy G. Westberg, Scott P. Mooney, and C.W. Mitchell are all doctoral students in the Department of Psychology, Indiana State University.

Address correspondence to I. Michael Shuff, PhD, Department of Counseling, 1516 Statesman Towers West, Indiana State University, Terre Haute, IN 47809.

INTRODUCTION

The purposes of this study were to describe the characteristics of volunteers in an AIDS hospice and to compare them to a group of volunteers from a traditional hospice. The AIDS volunteers came from Omega House in Houston, TX, founded in 1986 as one of the world's first AIDS dedicated residential hospices. The traditional hospice volunteers were drawn from New Age Hospice also located in Houston.

LITERATURE REVIEW

The social science literature that has mushroomed in the area of AIDS has focused largely on persons with AIDS, their families and friends. Volunteers in AIDS service organizations have commanded very little research attention. This review highlights the small body of literature on the characteristics of traditional hospice volunteers and the even smaller one on volunteers in AIDS service organizations.

Traditional Hospice Volunteers

A representative study of the early general hospice volunteers found the majority to be middle-aged, married women who had been college or university trained and who held strong religious beliefs (Caty & Tamlyn, 1983). In another study, the volunteers came from diverse work backgrounds, socioeconomic classes, and age groups, with students and retired persons forming an important basis of the group (Chng & Ramsey, 1984). Paradis and Usui (1987) noted a new trend in that more men were volunteering for hospice work. They attributed this specifically to the impact of AIDS on the gay community.

Patchner and Finn (1987-1988) surveyed general hospice volunteers with regard to characteristics, motivation, preparedness, satisfaction, and attitudes toward death. Their respondents felt well prepared to perform duties assigned to them and reported a high level of work satisfaction. In general, they valued most their direct contact with patients and families. A majority believed in life after death and occasionally thought about their own deaths. Only 9%

feared death, but a majority feared the pain associated with it. A majority also saw grief and mourning rituals as very important. Eighty-eight percent had experienced the death of a significant other.

Another group of volunteers undergoing the stress of hospice work turned most frequently to themselves or to their clients for help, although they also sought help from peers, friends, and family (Garfield & Jenkins, 1981-1982). They reported that client contact most often produced a feeling of uplift. It has further been noted that a clearly defined purpose seemed to be a significant factor in volunteers' coping and that they had a preference for emotion focused over problem focused coping strategies (Folkman & Lazarus, 1980).

A significant positive relationship between death anxiety and generalized anxiety was reported among general hospice workers (Amenta & Weiner, 1981a) as was a negative relationship between death anxiety and the sense of purpose in life (Amenta & Weiner, 1981b). Amenta (1984) also found that hospice volunteers who persisted in volunteer service longer than those who dropped out scored higher on purpose in life and lower on death anxiety.

Although personality characteristics have not been found especially useful in predicting hospice volunteer work performance, several characteristics assumed necessary have emerged from the literature: compassion, high tolerance for ambiguity, ability to talk about dying, ability for introspection, self-confidence, tolerance for frustration, psychological mindedness, humility, ability to speak in and understand metaphors, moderate to low levels of death anxiety, an element of spirituality, and relevant professional training (Paradis & Usui, 1987).

AIDS Program Volunteers

Williams (1988) surveyed volunteers in an AIDS Buddy Support program. The majority wanted to help specifically with AIDS patients while fewer simply wanted to be linked in some way with the gay community. The most disappointing aspect of volunteering to these subjects was the quality of relationship with the client which seemed to stem from personality differences and poor matches between buddy and client.

METHODS

Sample

The subjects in this study were 60 trained volunteers from Omega House and 40 from the New Age Hospice. Eighty percent of the active volunteers in each agency participated.

Instruments

We selected or designed instruments that would provide as relevant a profile as possible of the volunteers and the nature of their involvement. We chose materials from the areas of demographics, personality type, coping, and perceived threat. Perceived threat, a dimension not previously reported, seemed to figure prominently in the experience of volunteers that the senior author observed while at Omega House. For a full description of the rationale for instrument selection or development and issues concerning reliability and validity see Shuff (1989).

The Informational Questionnaire. The Informational Questionnaire, a 20-item, self-administered questionnaire, probes for pertinent demographic data. It also asks open-ended experiential questions about the volunteers' service such as its rewards and disappointments and the importance of spirituality in their lives.

The Myers-Briggs Type Indicator. The Myers-Briggs Type Indicator Form F is a 166-item, forced-choice, self-report inventory purporting to measure stable traits of personality style. It yields scores on four continuums: extroversion vs. introversion, sensing vs. intuition, thinking vs. feeling, and judging vs. perception. The Myers-Briggs Type Indicator is one of the most widely researched and used personality inventories available today (Carskadon, 1983). It is well-based in theory and is supported by a wealth of research (Willis, 1984).

The Ways of Coping Checklist. The Ways of Coping Checklist is a 66-item checklist describing a broad range of coping strategies people use in response to specific stressful situations. The instrument, a process not a trait measure, was designed to operationalize the theory of coping developed by Lazarus and his colleagues (Lazarus, 1966; Lazarus & Launier, 1978). Two empirically derived scales were used for this study: Problem Focused and Emotion Focused coping (Folkman & Lazarus, 1980).

The Spielberger State-Trait Anxiety Scale. We also administered the Spielberger State-Trait Anxiety Inventory (S-TAI). This 20-item self-report scale is considered among the best of the standardized anxiety measures (Dreger, in Buros, 1978).

The Perceived Threat Scale. The Perceived Threat Scale, a five item instrument developed especially for this study, asks the respondent to rate, on a four-point scale the threat he or she feels in five areas associated with hospice volunteer work: Physical Health, Social World, Employment, Emotional Health, and Total Threat.

Table 1 illustrates the intercorrelations of the subscales of the Perceived Threat Scale. There are modest but significant correlations among all of the subscales except for Emotional Health. Threats to Emotional Health, however, does correlate significantly with Total Threat, which is not assumed to be additive. The intercorrelations would seem to indicate that the scale is measuring variations on a common underlying construct.

Data Collection

Participation by volunteers was voluntary and anonymous. We collected data in the spring of 1988. Following the distribution of questionnaires, we made follow-up phone calls to insure a high return rate. In cases where missing data proved to be a problem, we substituted the mean value of the group's response to that item for the missing value (Tabachnick & Fidell, 1983). In cases in which too many data were missing to perform reliable statistical tests, we eliminated the records.

RESULTS AND DISCUSSION

Characteristics of the Groups

The New Age Hospice volunteers tended to be more homogeneous with regard to age, gender, sexual orientation, and previous volunteer experience than those from Omega House. They also

TABLE 1

SUBSCALE INTERCORRELATIONS (PEARSON r's)
PERCEIVED THREAT SCALE

N=76

	Health	Social World	Employment	Emotional Health	Total Threat
Health	1.000				
Social World	.295*	1.000			
Employment	.325*	.505*	1.000		
Emotional Health	.165	.134	.060	1.000	
Total Threat	.483*	.526*	.596*	.495*	1.000

* P < .05

tended to be more similar to other volunteer samples from traditional hospice programs in that they were middle-aged women with some previous personal experience with the loss of a close relative or friend to cancer (Caty & Tamlyn, 1983). They considered spirituality very to extremely important in their lives and they had moderate to low levels of anxiety. (See Table 5.) In comparison, the Omega House volunteers were a more diverse group on almost every demographic measure: age, gender, sexual orientation, occupation, and prior volunteer experience. They considered spirituality less important in their lives and had lower state-trait anxiety scores. Demographic and experiential data are presented in Table 2.

The MANOVA that we performed to isolate the demographic and experiential differences between the two groups was statistically significant. (See Table 3.) Of 16 demographic and experiential variables, eight differed significantly.

Gender. Gender significantly differentiated the two groups. New Age Hospice volunteers were predominantly female, those from Omega House mainly male. There was, however, a more even distribution of males and females at Omega House. This is consistent with recent hospice experience. As AIDS has made inroads into the population more males are becoming involved in hospice volunteering (Paradis & Usui, 1987).

Age. There was also a significant age difference between the two groups. Omega House volunteers were younger by a decade. In terms of gender and age the New Age subjects, were similar to those reported in the general hospice literature.

Employment. The two groups differed significantly in employment with New Age volunteers more homogeneous in their employment and Omega House volunteers gainfully employed and in a wider variety of occupations. This is understandable when one considers that 34% of New Age volunteers were either homemakers or retired. The range of occupational diversity at Omega House tended to act as a suppressor of the group's mean.

Sexual orientation. The greatest statistical difference found between the volunteers of the two hospices was that of sexual orientation. Ninety-five percent of New Age Hospice volunteers reported a heterosexual orientation, with 5% not responding to the question. On the other hand, 63% of Omega House volunteers reported themselves to be either homosexual or bisexual. The Omega House vol-

TABLE 2

SAMPLE CHARACTERISTICS

	Omega House N=60	New Age Hospice N=40
Gender: Male	63.3%	17.5%
Female	36.7%	82.5%
Age: Range	20.0-68.0	28.0-75.0
Mean	38.8	50.2
MDN	39.0	48.0
Mode	44.0	36.0
S D	10.3	13.1
Occupation:		
Management/Prof	44.1%	18.4%
Tech/Service	20.3%	31.6%
Teaching	5.1%	7.9%
Arts	6.8%	0.0%
Homemaker	3.4%	23.7%
Business	11.9%	7.9%
Student	5.1%	0.0%
Retired	3.4%	10.5%

92

Highest level of education completed:

High School	11.7%	15.0%
Tech/Trade School	3.3%	5.0%
College	38.8%	45.0%
Grad/Prof School	35.0%	20.0%
Postgrad School	11.7%	15.0%

Sexual orientation:

Heterosexual	36.7%	95.0%
Gay	58.3%	0.0%
Bisexual	5.0%	0.0%
No Response	0.0%	5.0%

Yearly income:

< $10,000	3.4%	5.3%
$10,000—$19,999	5.1%	18.4%
$20,000—$29,999	39.0%	13.2%
$30,000—$39,999	23.7%	18.4%
$40,000—$49,999	11.9%	21.1%
> $50,000	16.9%	23.7%

Present living circumstances:

Alone	40.0%	35.9%
With Parents	1.7%	0.0%
With Lover	21.7%	2.6%
With Spouse	20.0%	56.4%
With Roommate	15.0%	2.6%
Other	1.7%	2.6%

Table 2 (continued)

Length of hospice volunteering in months:

Range	1.0-27.0	2.0-84.0
Mean	9.85	20.97
MDN	10.00	20.00
Mode	12.00	4.00
S D	6.00	17.85

Previous volunteer experience:

Yes	67.7%	80.0%
No	38.8%	20.0%

Hospice volunteering differ from previous volunteer experience?

Yes	56.7%	82.1%
No	43.3%	17.9%

Major life change(s) within past six months:

Yes	38.3%	35.0%
No	61.7%	65.0%

Life affected by hospice volunteering:

Yes	93.3%
No	6.7%

Plans to continue hospice volunteering:

Yes	96.7%
No	3.3%

Prior experience with AIDS:

Yes	53.3%
No	46.7%

Prior experience with the terminally ill:

Yes	41.7%
No	58.3%

Importance of spirituality:

Not at All	11.7%
Somewhat	21.7%
Very	35.0%
Extremely	31.7%
Mean	1.87
MDN	2.00
S D	1.00

TABLE 3

MEANS, STANDARD DEVIATIONS, WILKS' LAMBDA, AND
UNIVARIATE F-TESTS
DEMOGRAPHIC AND EXPERIENTIAL VARIABLES

Variable	Omega House N = 54		New Age Hospice N = 29		Wilks' Lambda	F
	Mean	S. D.	Mean	S. D.		
Gender	1.370	.487	1.828	.384	.809	19.096*
Age	39.093	10.171	48.448	12.702	.858	13.377*
Employment	2.667	2.101	3.724	2.298	.948	4.476*
Education	4.241	1.098	4.276	.960	.999	.021
Sexual Orientation	1.704	.571	1.000	.000	.649	43.849*
Yearly Income	3.907	1.336	4.345	1.446	.977	1.910
Living Circumstances	2.759	1.636	2.655	1.542	.999	.079
Length Volunteered	9.482	5.287	19.517	19.650	.866	12.521*

Volunteered Before	1.370	.487	1.138	.351	.940	5.147*
Hospice Vol. Differing	1.426	.499	1.138	.351	.914	7.612*
Life Change	1.591	.500	1.621	.494	.999	.061
Life Affected	1.056	.231	1.034	.186	.998	.178
Continue Volunteering	1.037	.191	1.035	.186	.999	.004
AIDS Experience	1.444	.502	1.793	.412	.888	10.269*
Experience with Terminally Ill	1.574	.499	1.448	.506	.986	1.187
Spirituality	1.907	.996	2.276	.841	.966	2.869

(df = 1, 81)
*$P < .05$

unteers would seem to be more open about their sexuality in that none omitted answering this question.

Judging from responses to the open-ended questions on the Informational Questionnaire, differences in sexual orientation would seem to underlie, and thus might explain, the majority of differences observed between the two groups. Most of the volunteers came to each group following some personal encounter with death. This was especially true for the Omega House volunteers. They expressed a deep commitment to the gay community as a result of the AIDS epidemic. They regularly made references to repaying "the [gay] community." New Age volunteers were much more likely to have been motivated by a death from cancer. They did not with any frequency refer to any special community.

Length of time as a volunteer. Length of time volunteered also significantly differentiated the two groups. New Age Hospice volunteers tended to have volunteered at the hospice much longer than those at Omega House. Several factors that might account for this could have been at work. New Age Hospice had been in operation much longer than Omega House, thus there was simply not the opportunity for Omega House volunteers to have served any longer than 24 months. Since retired persons have more discretionary time, the older average age of New Age Hospice volunteers may also have accounted for some of their length of service. In addition, the effect of AIDS among the living on the personal lives of Omega House volunteers was sometimes a powerful determinant. As friends and lovers were diagnosed, the volunteers would frequently be forced by personal commitments to discontinue service.

Previous experience as a volunteer. New Age volunteers were significantly more likely to have done volunteer work previously than Omega House volunteers and these experiences were more diverse. They also viewed hospice volunteering as differing greatly from their past volunteer activities, again more so than Omega House volunteers. The age and occupational homogeneity factors were probably at work in these differences as well. AIDS service organization work tended to be the first volunteer experience for Omega House volunteers. Hospice experience would differ less markedly from this type of volunteering, since AIDS service volunteering also deals with the dying, than from other types of community service.

Prior experience with AIDS. The last of the demographic and experiential variables that produced a significant difference between the two groups was prior experience with AIDS. Not surprisingly, Omega House volunteers had much more.

Perceived Threat, Personality Type, and Ways of Coping

The MANOVA we performed to determine overall group differences in terms of perceived threat, personality type, and ways of coping revealed a statistically significant difference between the two groups. These results and those of the univariate F tests we conducted to isolate the specific differences between them appear in Table 4.

Perceived threat. Although the two groups did not differ on personality variables, personality type, or ways of coping, they did on four of the five subscales of the Perceived Threat to Health, Threat to Social World, Threat to Employment, and Total Threat. These significant differences are not surprising. New Age Hospice volunteers work in a socially sanctioned and community supported setting. What they do may not be understood but it is generally accorded at least lip service respect and admiration.

Omega House volunteers had every reason to expect just the opposite. The political climate in Houston at the time the study was conducted was homophobic and AIDS was considered a "gay plague" (Shilts, 1987). Various volunteers had had difficulties with family, friends, and the work setting in the course of their service and this was generally known among them all. Some volunteers felt more vulnerable than others. The degree of vulnerability seemed to relate to past experience, whether they had worked before with AIDS service organizations, whether they were gay, whether they were known and accepted at home and work given their sexual orientation, and whether they suspected that they might already be infected, or living among the ranks of the "worried well."

That threat to employment produced a significant difference between the two groups is understandable when one recalls that 34% of the New Age volunteers were either homemakers or retired. The Omega House volunteers were much more likely to have gainful

TABLE 4

MEANS, STANDARD DEVIATIONS, WILKS' LAMBDA, AND UNIVARIATE F-TESTS PERSONALITY RELATED VARIABLES

Variable	OMEGA HOUSE N = 48		NEW AGE HOSPICE N = 28		Wilks' Lambda	F
	Mean	S. D.	Mean	S. D.		
Extraversion–Introversion	97.250	28.054	99.107	23.721	.999	.087
Sensing–Intuition	107.292	27.988	111.321	27.645	.995	.370
Thinking–Feeling	109.979	20.495	112.107	19.128	.997	.200
Judging–Perceiving	97.583	27.775	102.536	28.100	.993	.557

Threats to:						
Health	.750	.636	.071	.262	.719	8.890*
Social World	.875	.959	.179	.476	.852	12.359*
Employment	.875	1.160	.000	.000	.824	15.841*
Emotional Health	.688	.719	.393	.497	.953	3.666
Total Threat	.792	.651	.143	.356	.758	23.597*
Problem Focused Coping	21.354	12.003	22.536	11.915	.998	.172
Emotionl Focused Coping	35.896	16.602	34.321	18.501	.998	.146

(df = 1, 74)
*P < .05

employment that might be taken from them should the nature of their volunteer work be known.

Personality type. Results of the Myers-Briggs Type Indicator revealed that both Omega House and New Age Hospice volunteers scored, as groups, close to the mean norm for the population of 100 on all four scales. The very slight variations of their scores from the normal puts both groups on the slightly more extroverted, intuitive, and feeling side. The New Age people might be considered a little perceiving or more comfortable living with open-endedness. These people like to wait for a great deal of information to be available before making decisions. The Omega volunteers, a shade more judging, would want to finish or settle with an issue sooner and then move on.

Ways of coping. Two subscales from the Ways of Coping Checklist were used in this study. The P scale is composed of problem focused coping strategies, the E of emotion focused ones. Both groups of volunteers reported relying more on emotion focused coping in dealing with stressful situations encountered in their hospice work.

It might have been expected that since Omega House volunteers' main job is to provide direct bedside and physical care that they would rely more on problem focused coping strategies. This was not, however, the case. Most of the stressful situations reported by both groups were not the sort to lend themselves to problem solving, action oriented strategies. Rather, all of the volunteers had to focus within themselves to adjust to extreme and unalterable situations. Examples they gave were a death scene, a grieving friend or inconsolable relative. The nature of this aspect of the volunteer work with the dying, no matter what the diagnosis, lends itself to reliance on emotion focused coping. This observation coupled with the finding that both groups are slightly more feeling types on the Myers-Briggs inventory would tend to outweigh any differences in specific patient care tasks that might have differentiated them.

Summary

The general finding that permeated all the results centered around the relative homogeneity of the New Age volunteers contrasted with the diversity of those from Omega House. The demographic and experiential profile of the New Age volunteers was much like that reported in other studies of hospice volunteers. Omega House volunteers did not fit that mold. They were more diverse in terms of age, sexual orientation, gender, and employment. They perceived themselves to be functioning under a moderate amount of threat to health, employment, social world, and threat in general (see Table 5).

POST HOC ANALYSIS

Since sexual orientation significantly differentiated the two groups and we wondered to what extent there might be differences in personality type, perceived threat, and ways of coping if we controlled for sexual orientation and matched for gender, we performed a post hoc analysis. We matched 18 heterosexually oriented participants from each hospice for gender and performed Student t tests on the following variables: spirituality, the four scales of the Myers-Briggs Type Indicator, the two scales of the State-Trait Anxiety Scale, the five scales of the Perceived Threat Scale, and the P and E scales of the Ways of Coping Checklist. The results are presented in Table 5.

Results

The two groups of heterosexual volunteers differed statistically on four of the 14 dimensions. They differed on perceived threats to health, to social world, to employment, and total threat. They did not differ on personality type, spirituality, anxiety, or coping style. It would appear that threats imposed by the nature of Omega House's mission to those dying of AIDS produced a significant amount of threat which distinguished between the two groups of volunteers. This perception of threat extended to the heterosexual volunteers of Omega House even though they did not fall into an epidemiological risk group for AIDS and in spite of the education given during their volunteer training aimed at ameliorating unrealistic fears.

TABLE 5
COMPARISON OF HETEROSEXUAL VOLUNTEERS
MEANS, STANDARD DEVIATIONS, AND t VALUES
SELECT PERSONALITY RELATED AND EXPERIENTIAL VARIABLES

	Omega House N = 18		New Age Hospice N = 18		
	Mean	S.D.	Mean	S.D.	t
Spirituality	1.890	.963	2.389	.850	1.539
Extraversion– Introversion	93.223	22.592	100.534	24.616	.970
Sensing– Intuition	115.110	24.034	125.000	57.638	.137
Thinking– Feeling	117.226	18.129	111.613	16.778	1.028
Judging– Perceiving	95.556	26.120	101.500	28.059	-.624
State Anxiety	31.777	7.623	37.278	8.478	.895
Trait Anxiety	34.667	9.160	38.294	7.016	1.749
Threat to Health	.611	.608	.056	.236	3.249*

Threat to Soc. World	.667	.767	.167	.383	2.404*
Threat to Employment	.556	.922	.000	.000	2.480*
Threat to Emo. Health	.944	.639	.444	.511	1.888
Total Threat	.833	.618	.167	.383	4.630*
Problem Focused	21.500	11.668	19.778	11.760	.607
Emotion Focused	39.611	18.324	31.389	17.030	1.382

(df = 17)
$p < .05$
Participants were matched for gender.

CONCLUSIONS AND RECOMMENDATIONS

This study sought to identify the uniqueness of the Omega House group by describing differences between the groups and it sought to identify the characteristics that uniquely characterized each group. Further research is indicated for perceived threat, as an aspect of the stress-coping paradigm as a construct worth further theoretical formulation and investigation.

Following the leads presented in this study, further research is also called for to describe more specifically the motivation of volunteers in an AIDS hospice. The AIDS hospice volunteers in spite of wide-ranging demographic differences form a cohesive group. They give the impression the group would not exist without an overwhelming outside circumstance to bring it and to keep it together. Understanding motivational and group process issues and how they affect each other might assist in bridging similar gaps in understanding that occur with other alienated groups.

AIDS hospice volunteer training and support programs should take into account the diversity of volunteers attracted to hospice service. Specific attention should be given to the large intragroup differences and provision should be made for including a variety of lifestyles.

Volunteer training in the AIDS hospice setting should assist volunteers in anticipating the threats they may encounter. It should help them to formulate a personalized coping style and plan to deal with the threats (Meichenbaum, 1977). To quote a volunteer, "Each learns to cope with death in his own way." There is a certain power in being able to predict stressful situations in advance and to develop a pre-need coping plan. This could be done if a careful inventory were developed of threatening situations typically encountered.

REFERENCES

Amenta, M. M. (1984). Death anxiety, purpose in life and duration of service in hospice volunteers. *Psychological Reports, 54,* 979-984.

Amenta, M. M., & Weiner, A. W. (1981a). Death anxiety and general anxiety in hospice work. *Psychological Reports, 49,* 962.

Amenta, M. M., & Weiner, A. W. (1981b). Death anxiety and purpose in life in hospice workers. *Psychological Reports, 49*, 920.

Carskadon, T. G. (ed.). (1983). *Research in Psychological Type.*

Caty, S., & Tamlyn, D. (1983). Hospice volunteers: a recruitment profile. *Dimensions in Health Service, 60*, 6, 22, 23.

Chng, C. L., & Ramsey, M. K. (1984-85). Volunteers and the care of the terminal patient. *Omega, 15*, 3, 237-244.

Dreger, R. Review of the State-Trait Anxiety Inventory. In O. Buros (Ed.), *The eighth mental measurements yearbook.* Highland Park, NJ: Gryphon Press, 1978, p. 1094.

Folkman, S., & Lazarus, R. S. (1980). An analysis of coping in a middle-aged community sample. *Journal of Health and Social Behavior, 21*, 219-239.

Garfield, C. A., & Jenkins, G. J. (1981-1982). Stress and coping of volunteers counseling the dying and bereaved. *Omega, 12*, 1-13.

Lazarus, R. S. (1966). *Psychological Stress and the Coping Process.* New York: McGraw-Hill.

Lazarus, R. S., & Launier, R. (1978). Stress-related transactions between person and environment. In Pervin, L. A. and Lewis, M. (eds.). *Perspectives in Interactional Psychology.* New York: Plenum.

Meichenbaum, D. (1977). *Cognitive-Behavior Modification: An Integrative Approach.* New York: Plenum.

Paradis, L. F., & Usui, W. M. (1987). Hospice volunteers: the impact of personality characteristics on retention and job performance. *The Hospice Journal, 3*, 1, 3-30.

Patchner, M. A., & Finn, M. B. (1987-1988). Volunteers: the life-line of hospice. *Omega, 18*, 2, 135-144.

Shilts, R. (1987). *And the Band Played On: Politics, People, and the AIDS Epidemic,* New York: St. Martin's Press.

Shuff, I. M. (1989). Volunteers functioning under threat: A comparison of AIDS hospice volunteers with general hospice volunteers. Unpublished doctoral dissertation, Indiana State University, Terre Haute.

Tabachnick, B. B., & Fidell, L. S. (1983). *Using Multivariate Statistics.* New York: Harper & Row.

Williams, M. J. (1988). Gay men as "buddies" to persons living with AIDS and ARC. *Smith College Studies in Social Work, 59*, 1, 38-52.

Willis, C. G. (1984). Myers-Briggs Type Indicator. In Keyser, D. J. and Sweetland, R. C. (eds.). *Test Critiques,* Vol. I. Kansas City: Test Corporation of America.

AIDS:
Experiences and Attitudes of Nurses from Rural Communities in Pennsylvania and New York

Deborah Bray Preston
Patricia Barthalow Koch
Elaine Wilson Young

SUMMARY. In this study we determined rural nurses' educational preparation concerning AIDS, whether they thought their health care facilities and communities were prepared to care for persons with AIDS, their attitudes toward AIDS and homosexuality, and in what ways AIDS had or might affect their practice. A questionnaire, which included the Nurses' AIDS Attitude Scale (NAAS), was administered to 738 employed registered nurses in 9 rural counties in Pennsylvania and New York. Findings suggest that this sample held many negative attitudes towards AIDS and homosexuality and had specific educational needs, especially in the psychosocial domain. They thought rural physicians and health care facilities were not yet well prepared to care for persons with AIDS.

INTRODUCTION

To date, AIDS has been largely confined to major metropolitan areas. It was estimated in 1986, however, that by 1991, 80% of the 145,000 people needing care for AIDS would be outside of New

Deborah Bray Preston, RN, PhD, is Assistant Professor of Health Education and Nursing, College of Health and Human Development, The Pennsylvania State University. Patricia Barthalow Koch, PhD, is Assistant Professor of Education; and Elaine Wilson Young, RN, PhD, is Adjunct Assistant Professor of Nursing at the same institution.

Address correspondence to Deborah Bray Preston, RN, PhD, College of Health and Human Development, The Pennsylvania State University, University Park, PA 16802.

York City and San Francisco, where 40% of all known AIDS patients were then being treated (CDC, 1986). More and more persons with AIDS are returning to their families of origin for support and care as their disease progresses (Burda, 1986; Graham & Cates, 1987; Levine, 1987; Rounds, 1988). Many of these families live in rural areas and if their sons developed AIDS through homosexual contact, they were probably not previously consciously aware of their sexual orientation (Rounds, 1988). This presents major problems since rural society is known to hold more conservative values with regard to sexuality (Larson, 1978). The expression of these conservative values has been evident in many parts of the country where persons with AIDS have been treated with discrimination, ostracism, homophobia, prejudice, and outright violence (Levine & Joyce, 1985).

Although educational programs, designed to clarify myths about AIDS and to help people handle their feelings and fears, have been shown to be helpful for those dealing with these issues, few are available in rural areas (Sontag, 1978). In addition, rural people are slower in adopting new ideas and are known to resist change more stubbornly than those in urban areas (Dillman & Hobbs, 1982). Another problem that may affect this public health crisis is the inadequacy of numbers of available health care facilities, health professionals, and health programs in nonmetropolitan parts of the country (Miller, 1982).

For these reasons and because privacy and anonymity are difficult to maintain in rural areas, persons with AIDS and their families may have to deal with a variety of problems that either do not affect, or vary in degree, from those of their urban counterparts. Because of the high prevalence of AIDS in the northeastern United States, these problems may be even more exaggerated in rural communities in this region.

A significant source of support for people with problems associated with AIDS is the professional nurse. Of all health care professionals, nurses come into the most regular, intimate, and prolonged contact with persons with AIDS (O'Donnell, O'Donnell, & Pleck, 1987; Young, Koch, & Preston, 1989). Moreover, nurses constitute the largest group of health service providers in rural communities, where they have been called specialists at being generalists. They practice in a variety of settings rather than exclusively in specialty areas and they often work independently due to geographic isolation and scarcity of physicians and organized health care facilities (Lassiter, 1985).

As members of the community, rural nurses are acutely aware of local health care problems and, even if not formally employed, they are often sought out for information and for help (Lassiter, 1985). It is safe, therefore, to say that they will be the professionals managing the bulk of care for persons with AIDS and their families in inpatient facilities, community settings, and at home. They will be looked to as sources of health education and health programming in schools, the workplace, and clinics. Because of the information lag to rural areas and the prevalence of conservative values, it is anticipated that rural nurses are already having, or will soon have, even more difficulty dealing with AIDS than their urban-based colleagues.

In some parts of the country nurses are already refusing to care for AIDS patients because of the nurses' fear of the disease and its transmissibility as well as their discomfort with homosexuality (Frank, 1986; Nelson, Maxey, & Keith, 1984). Studies have shown that nurses in general not only need technical information about AIDS, but also help in dealing with their feelings towards homosexuality if they are to adequately care for these patients (van Servellen, Lewis, & Leake, 1988; Young, 1988; Young et al., 1989). Thus, unless nurses have sufficient educational preparation and develop nonjudgmental attitudes, i.e., lack of fear of and discomfort with AIDS and homosexuality, care for persons with AIDS and their families will suffer. To our knowledge there are no research studies that document the extent to which AIDS has affected rural nursing practice.

THE STUDY

Purpose

The purpose of this study was to determine what educational preparation rural nurses have had about AIDS, whether or not they felt that the health care facilities in their communities were prepared to care for people with AIDS, their attitudes towards AIDS and homosexuality, and in what ways AIDS had or might affect their practice.

METHODS

Site Selection

We collected data as part of the larger "Nursing and AIDS: A Rural Perspective" project funded by the United States Department of Agriculture through the Northeast Regional Center for Rural Development. The study sites were seven rural counties in Pennsylvania and two in New York, all chosen on the basis of rural population as a substantial proportion of total population. In Pennsylvania where the total population is 30.7% rural, counties range from 100% rural to 2.9% rural. The seven counties in the study have rural populations of 90% and above and all lie outside of Metropolitan Statistical Areas (MSAs) (U.S. Bureau of Census, 1981). We chose the counties in New York through a topology of New York State counties that identifies extent of urban influence (Eberts, 1984). Seven of New York's 44 counties have been classified as limited in urban influence based on: the extent to which people live in communities of less than 2,500; the size of the largest community in the county; and the extent to which people commute outside the county for employment. Using these criteria we chose two of the most rural.

The Sample

We purchased the lists of all licensed registered nurses living in these nine counties from the Bureau of Professional and Occupational Affairs in Pennsylvania (N = 1009) and from the Division of Professional Licensing Service in New York State (N = 1016). Because these lists do not indicate employment status, we mailed questionnaires to everyone whose name was on the lists (N = 2025). We sent a follow-up postcard three weeks later. A month after that we sent a second questionnaire to which 1073 or 53% of the nurses responded. Of those finally returned 962 (89.9%) were usable for data analysis. Seven hundred thirty-eight of these nurses or 76.7% of the total sample were currently employed in nursing. These 738 respondents constituted the study sample.

Instrumentation

In addition to demographic items, the questionnaire contained sections assessing nurses' knowledge, professional practices, and attitudes related to AIDS. The Nurses' AIDS Attitude Scale (NAAS), the instrument used in this study, contains 39 attitudinal statements to which the subject can respond on a Likert scale from "1" – "strongly agree" to "5" – "strongly disagree" with the midpoint representing "neither agree nor disagree" (Preston, Young, & Koch, 1990). Principal axis factor analysis (PA $_2$) using a varimax rotation has established three factors in this scale explaining 41% of the variance. Factor 1 (caring for persons with AIDS/ contact issues) and Factor 2 (knowing HIV status) statements are contained within Part 1 of the NAAS, whereas Factor 3 (homosexuality) statements are found in Part 2. Internal consistency of the NAAS has been established at .95 using Cronbach's alpha coefficient of reliability.

A higher score on the NAAS indicates more positive attitudes towards AIDS-related issues, whereas a lower score indicates negative attitudes towards AIDS and homosexuality. In addition, questions were asked about: (1) access to AIDS education; (2) additional information they felt they needed; (3) how well-prepared they felt to care for persons with AIDS; (4) how well-prepared they felt their communities were to care for persons with AIDS; and (5) what their practice regarding AIDS presently was or had been.

RESULTS

Description of the Sample

The respondents were overwhelmingly female between the ages of 21 and 65 years of age (see Tables 1 and 2). Most were white and 594 (81.9%) were married. Seventy-one percent stated they were educated in diploma or associate degree programs while 23 % were bachelors prepared either in nursing or another field. Approximately 6% had graduate degrees. Fifty-one and seven-tenths percent practiced in hospitals and 17.2% in community health. Most were staff nurses (57.4%) with 24.2% working in management positions.

Table 1

Description of the Sample of Rural Nurses
N=738

	n	Percent
Gender		
Female	714	97.5
Male	18	2.5
*Missing	6	
Age		
<25	34	4.7
25-29	63	8.7
30-49	469	65.0
50-64	146	20.2
>65	10	1.4
*Missing	16	
Race		
White	720	98.5
Other	11	1.5
*Missing	7	
Marital Status		
Single	131	18.1
Married	594	81.9
*Missing	13	
Education		
Diploma	307	41.8
Associate Degree	214	29.1
B.S. in Nursing	117	15.9
B.S. in Other Field	52	7.1
Graduate	45	6.1
*Missing	3	

*Percentages calculated on reported data.

Rural Nurses' Educational Preparation for AIDS

Table 3 illustrates the sources of AIDS education reported by the sample. Nursing and inservice education were the most frequently reported sources of information with other professional journals and commercial television programming the next most prevalent. Eighty-two percent of nurses in the sample reported having had education in AIDS transmission and contagion and 69% in infection policies and procedures while only 47% reported having had in-

Table 2

Employment Status of Rural Nurses
N=738

	n	Percent
Setting		
Hospital	375	51.7
Community Health	125	17.2
Ambulatory Care	37	5.1
Nursing Home	89	12.3
Industry	6	.8
School	70	9.7
Nursing Education	23	3.2
*Missing	13	
Position		
Staff Nurse	418	57.4
Clinical Specialist/		
Nurse Practitioner	17	2.3
Nurse Manager	84	11.5
Supervisor	92	12.7
Nurse Anesthetist	13	1.8
Educator	51	7.0
Other	53	7.3
*Missing	10	

*Percentages calculated on reported data.

struction in homosexuality and bisexuality. Fewer than 29% of the sample reported having had instruction in symptom control, psychological, spiritual, social, legal, and financial needs of families of persons with AIDS, or hospice care. In addition, only 16% reported having been taught how to manage their own psychological needs when dealing with AIDS patients.

Preparation of Community Health Care Systems for AIDS

Subjects were asked how well they felt they were prepared to care for persons with AIDS, how well they felt the physicians in their communities were prepared, and how well they felt the health care facilities in their communities were capable of meeting the AIDS crisis (see Table 4). Eighteen percent felt well prepared, 65% felt somewhat prepared, and 17% did not feel well prepared. Six-

Table 3

Educational Preparation for AIDS
of Rural Nurses
N=738

	n	**Percent
Sources of AIDS Education		
Nursing Journals	436	60.0
Inservice Programs	390	53.6
Other Professional Journals	314	43.2
Television	277	38.1
Professional Workshops	258	35.5
Bulletins (e.g., CDC Publications)	211	29.0
Films/Videos	155	21.3
Professional Meetings	74	10.2
*Missing	11	
Had Instruction In		
Transmission & Contagion	596	82.0
Infection Policies & Procedures	502	69.1
Homosexuality & Bisexuality	341	46.9
Health Care Resources for AIDS	295	40.6
Providing Supportive Care Until Death	223	30.7
Psychological Needs of PWAs & Families	208	28.6
Symptoms Control	200	27.5
Spiritual Needs of PWAs & Families	166	22.8
Families Involvement in Care	162	22.3
Social Needs of PWAs & Families	158	21.7
Psychological Needs of Caregivers (nurses)	118	16.2
Financial Needs of PWAs & Families	58	8.0
Legal Needs of PWAs & Families	46	6.3
*Missing	11	

*Percentages calculated on reported data.
**Percentages do not total 100.
Subjects answered more than one question.

Table 4

Rural Nurses' Opinions About Preparation of Their
Community Health Care Systems to Care for Persons With AIDS
N=738

	Percentages		
	Well Prepared	Somewhat Prepared	Not Well Prepared
Subject's Own Preparation	17.6	65.0	17.4
Rural Community Physicians	15.9	65.4	18.7
Rural Community Health Care Facilities	13.2	59.4	27.4

teen percent felt the physicians in their communities were well prepared, 65% felt physicians were somewhat prepared, and 19% felt
they were not well prepared. Thirteen percent felt that the health
care facilities in their communities could presently meet the challenge of AIDS, 59% felt their facilities were somewhat prepared,
whereas 27% felt their communities were not well prepared. When
asked in an open-ended question whether or not they felt their employers were or would be supportive in carrying out universal precautions, 89% felt they would.

AIDS and Rural Nurses' Attitudes

The respondents' attitudes toward AIDS and homosexuality measured by the Nurses AIDS Attitude Scale (NAAS) are arrayed in
Tables 5 and 6 which also contain examples of statements on the
instrument. For purposes of clarity we used only the percentages of
respondents who neither agreed nor disagreed (were ambivalent),
agreed, or strongly agreed to illustrate the segment of the sample
that was concerned to phobic about AIDS and homonegative to homophobic about gay men. As indicated in Tables 5 and 6, percentages of nurses whose attitudes fell within these categories ranged

Table 5

Rural Nurses' Attitudes About AIDS
N=738

| | *Percentages | | |
Selected Statements	Ambivalent	Agree	Strongly Agree
Nurses should be able to refuse to care for PWAs.	15.6	18.3	4.8
I am bothered that I might not be able to prevent myself from contracting AIDS.	18.2	29.7	8.6
I feel worried about the possibility of acquiring AIDS from patients.	17.9	37.5	6.1
I feel angry about possibly caring for a PWAs who contracted the disease through high risk sexual behavior.	26.3	19.8	7.9
I am fearful of caring for PWAs because there is no cure.	20.3	33.4	8.9

*Each statement reflects the percentages of the 738 respondents. This table is not cumulative.

from 38.7 to 62.6 indicating more negative than positive attitudes towards AIDS and male homosexuality.

In an attempt to gain a more rounded sense of our subjects' attitudes, we asked several open-ended questions. The following statements characterize their concerns:

• I feel like my life and future are put in jeopardy.

• Our nurses would be afraid of these clients and many would refuse.

• AIDS patients are not common, yet each is treated like a leper. We also are not given the freedom of choice to care for these patients if we are not comfortable with them.

• We are probably more fearful because the sparse AIDS population makes it impractical to have one staff caring for AIDS patients alone — fear of transmitting the disease to other patients or myself by bouncing back and forth.

- I feel very sorry for persons who contract AIDS from transfusions, heredity, etc., but am very angry with those who contract AIDS by drug use, homosexuality, etc.

- To my knowledge, we have no AIDS patients in the community. General feeling of anyone in our area is "stay away from him." I would be very cautious.

- This is not a "high risk" area at present. Because of the limited education of many in this rural area, homosexuals and AIDS are shunned, feared, misunderstood, etc.

- We would be frightened if we knew we had an AIDS patient in our hospital.

- Each of our AIDS clients is in an isolated area. Some have no family or social support at all — getting them to needed treatment has been difficult — as providers become suspicious and refuse.

- Essentially a "redneck" county so if they were to appear in public places certain people would make life very difficult anyway. Were the person a homosexual on top of it, there just isn't any support or respect here for them. One client has to go 100 miles away to stay until he dies. No help here.

- AIDS has made nursing a "high risk" profession.

- I have never cared for an AIDS patient and I have had many of my nurses say they would not take care of a known AIDS patient. In all honesty, the whole idea of the HIV is frustrating as is my negative attitude of homosexuals.

AIDS and Rural Nurses' Practice

Forty-two percent of the respondents reported having cared for AIDS patients; most for only one or two (see Table 7). About 20% expressed a distinct unwillingness to care for persons with AIDS.

Table 7 lists the percentages of respondents willing to engage in specific nursing practices with a patient whose HIV status was

Table 6

Rural Nurses' Attitudes About Homosexuality
N=738

| | *Percentages | | |
Selected Statements	Ambivalent	Agree	Strongly Agree
Male homosexuality is obscene and vulgar.	39.3	26.0	13.7
Male homosexuality endangers the institution of the family.	22.2	35.1	16.3
I feel disgusted when I consider the state of sinfulness of male homosexuality.	35.8	22.1	9.9
Male homosexuality should be considered immoral.	25.3	21.4	12.7
I feel revolted when I think of two men engaged in private sexual behaviors with each other.	29.3	32.4	17.5

*Each statement reflects the percentages of the 738 respondents. This table is not cumulative.

known to be positive. When asked how others in their lives would feel about their caring for persons with AIDS, many felt that their lovers (60%), spouses (72%), parents (72%), and children (56%) would be slightly to extremely upset if they (the nurses) cared for persons with AIDS. In addition, many subjects responded with written statements. Some examples follow:

- If I were single without children, I would not be so reluctant to take care of an AIDS patient. In order for me to agree to take care of an AIDS patient, I would need to be convinced that the best precautions possible were being exercised.

- I quit one job because there were too many AIDS patients and I couldn't choose not to work with them all the time. I now have a job where I only occasionally work with known HIV positive patients.

- Depending on whether the patient was an innocent (baby, etc.)

or drug abuser or gay, my feeling and care would be determined.

• If I have a patient who is positive, I probably would refuse. I do not want to expose myself and my young children to the disease. No gowns, gloves, masks, etc., are 100% guaranteed to stop the virus spread. Until more research is done to establish that I would not get the disease, I would have to refuse.

• I may be prejudiced but any adult who contracted AIDS by sexual behavior deserves it. I feel sorry for anyone who has AIDS by no fault of their own. I also feel gays have a right to their lifestyle but I don't force my lifestyle on them and I resent them trying to force their lifestyle on me. As for their rights, what about our rights? They choose the way they live and I resent thinking I may get their disease because they need their rights. Lepers are isolated to protect other people and people with leprosy had no choice about getting it.

• As a group, homosexuals are too "touchy" about attitudes. There is too much emphasis on attitudes. I believe homosexuality is immoral but so are many other behaviors such as fornication, but it is rampant and everyone has the right to do what he (she) wants as long as it doesn't endanger others.

• We all know it is a sin. When they came out to demand their rights in government, God stepped in with AIDS. That's how I feel about it.

Many were more positive in tone:

• I'm thankful that our area has very few people touched by AIDS, but also feel confident that the AIDS patients we do encounter will be treated with respect and dignity and will receive skillful care. Compassion and empathy are essential in any area of nursing and our agency has plenty of both.

• With universal precautions, it will mostly be my own fault if I contract AIDS. Caring for AIDS patients is special just as is oncology nursing. You are helping a person to die in peace.

• I am not afraid of AIDS and nursing allows me to show the

patients with AIDS that they are not alone and not everyone fears them.

• It challenges our profession to better itself in regards to infection control, psychological care of the terminally ill, observation, and treatment skills, etc.

• When I care for AIDS patients, I don't feel I treat them any different than any other patient, only for the exception of implementing universal precautions.

DISCUSSION

This study serves as a foundation for understanding rural nursing attitudes and practice with regard to AIDS. Although only 42% of respondents in this sample reported having taken care of persons with AIDS, predictions are that the prevalence in rural areas will markedly increase. Thus, growing numbers of rural nurses will be called upon to become AIDS care providers (D'Augelli, 1989). At present there are fewer of them with experience than without.

Findings from this study indicated that this sample of rural nurses displayed many negative attitudes towards AIDS and homosexuality. Given the professional ethical mandate of nursing care set forth in the American Nurses Association Standards of Nursing Care, almost 20% expressed an unwillingness altogether to care for persons with AIDS as well as an unwillingness to provide specific nursing-care procedures to persons with AIDS. In addition, many reported that their families would be upset if they were to care for AIDS patients.

Further need for AIDS education was also indicated, particularly in the psychosocial aspects of the disease and the need for hospice-like supportive care. If these rural nurses' perceptions of community preparedness are correct, rural physicians and health care facilities are not yet well prepared to meet the mounting crisis and they too will need education and support.

Table 7

Variables Related to Nursing
Practice and AIDS
N=738

Behaviors	n	Missing	*Percent
Willing to care for PWAs			
Yes	580	17	80.4
No	141		19.6
Have cared for PWAs			
Yes	301	17	41.7
No	420		58.3
**Willing to:			
Provide physical comfort	683	14	94.3
Provide noninvasive nursing care	665	19	92.5
Talk to patient about I.V. drug use	648	12	89.3
Provide total nursing care including invasive procedures	496	20	69.1
Draw blood	450	21	62.8
Talk to patient about his sexual behavior	449	17	62.3
Perform mouth to mouth resuscitation with a tube	337	23	47.1
Perform mouth to mouth resuscitation without a tube	54	23	7.6

*Percentages are calculated on reported data
(N - missing values)

**Percentages do not total 100. Subjects answered more than one question.

RECOMMENDATIONS

These findings emphasize the need for continuing education programs for nurses and other rural health care workers that include the affective as well as the technical aspects of AIDS as well as the basics of hospice-like supportive care. The need to help nurses as well as their families deal with their negative feelings towards AIDS and homosexuality is also indicated.

REFERENCES

Burda, D. (1986, February 5). Specialty hospitals: Small and rural await the impending AIDS crisis. *Hospitals*, 71-72.

Center for Disease Control (1986, June 12). Press release.

Centers for Disease Control (1987). Human immunodeficiency virus infection in the United States. *Morbidity and Mortality Weekly Reports, 36*, Suppl. No. S-6.

Centers for Disease Control (1989). *HIV/AIDS Surveillance Report*, September, 1-16.

D'Augelli, A. R. (1989). AIDS fears and homophobia among rural nursing personnel. *AIDS Education and Prevention, 1*(4), 277-284.

Dillman, D., & Hobbs, D. (1982). *Rural society in the U.S.: Issues for the 1980's*. Boulder, CO: Westview Press.

Eberts, P.R. (1984). *Socioeconomic trends in rural New York State: Toward the twenty-first century*. State of New York, Legislative Commission on Rural Resources, Albany.

Frank, H. (1986). AIDS – The responsibility of health workers to assume some degree of personal risk. *The Western Journal of Medicine, 144*, 363-364.

Graham, L., & Cates, J. (1987). AIDS: Developing a primary health care task force. *Journal of Psychosocial Nursing, 25*(12), 21-25.

Larson, O. (1978). Values and beliefs of rural people. In T. Ford (Ed.). *Rural USA: Persistence and change*. Ames, IA: Iowa State University Press.

Lassiter, P. (1985). Education for rural health professionals: Nurses. *The Journal of Rural Health, 1*(1), 23-28.

Levine, C., & Joyce, B. (Eds.). (1985). AIDS: The emerging ethical dilemma. *Hastings Center Report Special Supplement*, 15:4, Hastings-on-Hudson, NY: Hastings Center.

Levine, R. (1987, December). What rural America needs to know about AIDS. *Healthlink*, 30-31.

Miller, M. K. (1982). Health and medical care. In D. Dillman & D. Hobbs (Eds.), *Rural Society in the U.S.: Issues for the 1980's*. Boulder, CO: Westview Press.

Nelson, W. J., Maxey, L., & Keith, S. (1984). Are we abandoning the AIDS patient? *RN, 6,* 18-19.

O'Donnell, L., O'Donnell, C. R., & Pleck, J. H. (1987). Psychosocial responses of hospital workers to acquired immune deficiency syndrome (AIDS). *Journal of Applied Social Psychology, 17*(3), 269-285.

Preston, D. B., Young, E. W., & Koch, P. B. (1990). Nurses' AIDS Attitude Scale (NAAS). Unpublished manuscript. The Pennsylvania State University, University Park, PA.

Rounds, K.A. (1988). AIDS in rural areas: Challenges to providing care. *Social Work, 33,* 257-261.

Sontag, S. (1978). *Illness as metaphor.* New York: Random House.

U.S. Bureau of Census. (1981). 1980 Census of Population. Washington, DC: USGPO.

Van Servellen, G., Lewis, C., & Leake, B. (1988). Nurses' responses to the AIDS crisis: Implications for continuing education programs. *The Journal of Continuing Education in Nursing, 19*(1), 4-8.

Young, E. W. (1988). Nurses attitudes toward homosexuality: Analysis of change in AIDS workshops. *Journal of Continuing Education in Nursing, 19*(1), 9-12.

Young, E. W., Koch, P. B., & Preston, D. B. (1989). AIDS and homosexuality: A longitudinal study of knowledge and attitude change among rural nurses. *Public Health Nursing, 6*(4), 189-196.

Dying in Prison:
Sociocultural
and Psychosocial Dynamics

Fleet Maull

SUMMARY. In January 1988, an inmate-staffed hospice volunteer program began operation at a federal correctional medical facility, with the goal of meeting the unique psychosocial, palliative, and spiritual needs of terminally ill prisoners, primarily men with AIDS and cancer. This paper discusses sociocultural and psychosocial characteristics of the incarcerated patients and the prison hospital setting. It presents a number of case examples. Particular attention is given to the effect that an environment of intensified anger, hostility, distrust, and despair has on the coping mechanisms of terminally ill, incarcerated patients.

Fleet W. Maull, MA, is a doctoral student in psychology at California Coast University, a member of the Hospice Volunteer Group at the US Medical Center for Federal Prisoners, and an instructor in the Medical Center's Adult Basic Education Program.

The author acknowledges the contributions of all the inmate volunteers, staff members, visiting community professionals, and patients to the Medical Center's Hospice Program and the review of an early draft of this article by a number of hospital staff members, inmate volunteers, and professional colleagues.

Address correspondence to the author at the US Medical Center, PO BOX 4000/19864-044, Springfield, MO 65808.

The views expressed in this paper are the author's own and do not represent in any way the official views or policies of the U.S. Medical Center for Federal Prisoners or the U.S. Bureau of Prisons. In the case examples the names of the patients and other nonessential details have been changed in order to protect the rights of privacy of the patients and their families. The examples, however, do accurately depict the issues and events of actual cases. They are neither composites nor in any way fictional.

INTRODUCTION

As of May 1989 in the United States nearly 628,000 men and women, more than the population of Milwaukee, were incarcerated in state and federal prisons. Another 150,000 filled the country's county jails to well beyond capacity. By 1993, the federal prison population is expected to increase by more than 75% from its 1989 level to 84,000 and state prison populations are expected to increase in similar proportions (Lacayo, 1989). Soon more than 1 million people over 16 years old will be incarcerated in the U. S.

With the move toward determinant (no-parole) sentencing, stiffer penalties for both first offenders and habitual offenders, and increasingly vigorous prosecution of those involved in drug trafficking and "white collar crime," the exponential growth in the prison population can be expected to continue indefinitely.

The normal incidence of death in this adult population is now increased because of the AIDS epidemic. From October 1987 to October 1989, National Institute of Justice figures indicate a 175% increase in the cumulative total of AIDS cases diagnosed among U.S. federal, state, and local prisoners — as compared to 163% in the population at large during the same period. The annual incidence rate of AIDS in the U.S. population was 14.6 cases per 100,000 in 1989, up from 13.3 in 1988. The aggregate incidence rate for all state and federal correctional systems was 202 per 100,000 in 1989, more than twice the 1988 rate. (National Institute of Justice, 1990). As of October 1988, AIDS had been diagnosed in 5,411 correctional inmates and 751 had died in custody (National Institute of Justice, 1990).

Until recently, the Parole Commission in the federal prison system had the option of sending some prisoners home to die; but with the move to determinant sentencing, the commission will no longer have this option. Many more men and women are dying in U. S. prisons than ever before. Inferring from the statistics just cited, it seems certain that this trend will continue through the present decade, creating a critical present and future need for palliative care at U. S. correctional medical facilities.

This paper examines the effects that incarceration and the prison hospital setting have on seriously ill and dying patients. It also delineates prisoners' unique psychosocial experiences and coping mechanisms observed by inmate volunteers working under the direction of staff professionals in a new hospice program at the U. S. Medical Center for Federal Prisoners begun in 1988 in Springfield, Missouri.

THE PRISON HOSPITAL SETTING

In discussing the principal objectives of palliative or hospice care, Zimmerman (1986) suggests that perhaps the term "graceful" rather than "dignified" is a better way to express "the way in which most of us wish to die" (pp. 6-7). Yet Clemmer (cited in Heffernan, 1972, p. 4), in a classic study of prison social organization, graphically describes the prison world as "graceless," a world of "drabness . . . monotony and stupor" where "trickery and dishonesty overshadow sympathy and cooperation." Thus, the challenge of a prison hospice program is to enhance the quality of life, and death, for prisoners dying in a completely *graceless* environment that inherently deprives them of their dignity as human beings.

The prison hospital setting is characterized by many limitations and constraints, with security the first priority, above even medical attention in importance. Many terminally ill prisoners feel isolated, helpless, angry, fearful, and sometimes hopeless. Although medical care at U.S. correctional facilities might be considered, at least by legal minimum standards, adequate and humane in most cases, patients and their families may perceive it as substandard, cruel, and inhumane (Kubler-Ross, 1987).

Prisoner/patients and their families have virtually no choice of primary care giver, treatment, or medication. Indeed, physicians in this setting often have limited options for treatment, and they usually are given limited time to attend to their patients. Hospice protocols for pain management are rare. Many prison staff physicians, afraid of encouraging drug abuse or addiction, are extremely conservative in prescribing narcotics, even to dying patients.

The attitudes of the patients' primary care givers — physicians, nurses, and ward correctional officers — vary from benevolent and caring through degrees of professional decency to outright indifference and sometimes hostility. Staff who wish to give their patients optimal care often risk the resentment and suspicion of their colleagues when they do. As in traditional hospitals, the great majority of prison hospital nurses are women. In a men's prison female nurses who spend any more than the minimal time alone with their patients may suffer the suspicions and criticism of the ward correctional officer as well as some of their colleagues.

Patients who are weak or feeble or semiconscious from illness or medication often fear abuse by inmate nursing attendants and orderlies. They fear their watches, shoes, or anything else of value may be stolen. Some hospital workers even charge patients for the services they are supposed to provide as part of their duties and ignore or do the minimum for patients who will not or cannot pay. It is also common for inmate hospital workers to remove portions of meat, fruit, and desserts or other desirable items from patients' meal trays before serving them. Supervisors, too busy to notice or too concerned with retaining inmate-workers' services to investigate suspected abuses, do not confront the issue unless someone is caught in the act.

Further compromising the nutrition of inmate patients is the tendency for food to be of poor quality and served in an unappetizing fashion. While some institutions do make an effort to provide special diets and supplemental foods for their medical patients, diet limitations and the quality of food preparation are, nonetheless, a continual source of frustration and the cause of increased feelings of helplessness. When patients are very ill, uncomfortable, or in a lot of pain, it is very difficult to get them to eat foods they do not like or that they find unappetizing, even when they know their very survival depends on their eating well.

Prison patients' support systems are limited because incarceration restricts contacts with family and friends in several ways. Those in federal prison facilities are likely to be far from home, making it very expensive for loved ones to visit. Patients may also be isolated from their families due to either their own or their family's sense of shame or blame. Within the prison community itself, patients are often kept on locked wards where they are unable to go to the recreation yards for fresh air, participate in programs for education or recreation, or go to the prison chapel for religious services.

Even within the small world of a prison hospital ward, patients may be further isolated by the debilitating effects of their disease, by language barriers, by the fear of being abused by others, or, in the case of those with AIDS, by the fear that others have of their disease (Kubler-Ross, 1987). Although patients in other institutional care settings may share similar constraints, in the prison environment, pervaded by distrust, anger, and hostility, these conditions are significantly intensified.

THE PSYCHOSOCIAL IMPACT OF INCARCERATION

Loss and Grief,
the Prisoner's Bereavement Process

A prisoner's life, whether he is well or sick, is pervaded by loss: loss of freedom, loss of dignity, loss of former social or professional status, and, most critically, loss of the supportive environment provided by significant others. Many prisoners have experienced the complete disintegration of their families through divorce and lost custody of or visitation rights with their children. Many have also lost their real and personal assets, great or small. Simply put, many prisoner have lost almost everything that formerly gave their lives meaning.

Rando (1984) defines grief in part as "the reaction to many kinds of loss, not necessarily death alone" (p. 15), and cites 15 types of loss undergone by dying patients. All the dramatic losses experienced by most prisoners are included on this list. Prisoners have severe grief by virtue of incarceration alone. Rando also describes anticipatory grief, or grief for future losses. The prisoner told that he or she has a life-threatening illness grieves not only for all that has already been lost but for all that will be lost in death.

Social and Psychological Death
as a Result of Incarceration

Rando (1984, citing Sudnow) describes four stages that everyone goes through as he or she dies: social death, psychological death, biological death, and physiological death. Even healthy prisoners experience the first of these, "social death, . . . symbolic death of the [person] in the world the [person] has known (p. 207)." With the effects of a lengthy incarceration healthy prisoners often experience a degree of Sudnow's "psychological death" as well. They regress and become helpless and dependent. Many prisoners then, even without falling ill, are already undergoing, to one degree or another, these first two stages of death.

Parallels Between Kubler-Ross's Stages of Dying and the Adjustment to Incarceration

Inmate hospice volunteers uniformly report that their own experiences of adjusting to incarceration have been similar to the five stages of emotional reaction Kubler-Ross (1969) describes in terminally ill patients: denial and isolation, anger, bargaining, depression, and acceptance. The volunteers also report observing their fellow prisoners pass through the same steps.

New arrivals, fresh from trial and sentencing, typically deny. They simply cannot believe that the worst has happened, and they are convinced that their conviction will be overturned on appeal. They talk about being back on the street in a matter of weeks or months.

As appeals are lost and the reality of doing prison time sets in, denial turns to anger and often to depression. Bargaining with good behavior and program involvement for the hope of parole or some other sentence relief is commonly mixed with an underlying hostility toward the system and all those who represent it. The predominant emotions in the prison environment are pervasive anger and hostility mixed with — sometimes real, but more often false — hope for early reprieve. Though a few prisoners may move beyond the anger and the blaming toward a degree of healthy acceptance, self-responsibility, and growth, the vast majority remain angry and often bitter throughout.

PSYCHOSOCIAL EXPERIENCE AND COPING MECHANISMS OF TERMINALLY ILL PRISONER/PATIENTS

For prisoners a diagnosis of terminal illness compounds the underlying grief over the losses attendant to incarceration. Prison hospice volunteers regularly report behavior in their patients that resembles the coping mechanisms and patterns observed by Kubler-Ross (1969), Rando (1984), and others. Many factors, however, affect how patients cope with these stages in the prison setting.

Kelly (1988) notes that the emotions of a condemned man awaiting execution are similar to Kubler-Ross's (1969) five stages of death. Certainly there is little difference between telling a prisoner with more than 6 months to serve that he will die in less than 6 months and condemning him to await execution on death row. In fact, death row is exactly what the patients call the cancer ward.

From what we have seen as volunteers in the prison hospice program, a prison patient's first reaction to a diagnosis of terminal illness is usually shock, followed almost immediately by withdrawal and depression. Sometimes, patients appear to spin through the first four of Kubler-Ross's five stages in a matter of hours or days, but as the initial shock wears off, denial normally emerges as the predominant coping mechanism.

Denial: Coping with the Fear of Dying in Prison

Confronted by the likelihood of dying in prison, the patient's initial reaction of denial is perhaps the most useful defense against the onslaught of an overwhelming sense of fear, isolation, hopelessness, failure, and despair.

The denial process for incarcerated patients is reinforced by the almost universal belief that if they could get outside medical care they would not be dying. Therefore, prison hospice patients typically focus on the hope of a special medical parole, or some other form of early medical release, rather than on adjusting to the prospect of dying let alone dying in prison. Time and time again, hospice patients have stated in one way or another that death in prison is the ultimate failure in life, worse than all the others. It may or may not be true in general that no one really ever wants to die (Weisman, cited in Buschman, 1968), but it is almost certainly true that no one wants to die in prison.

Case Example — Paul

Paul, a prisoner in his late 40s, was admitted to the hospice program terminally ill with AIDS. When the hospice volunteer first visited him, Paul was receiving an intravenous blood plasma supplement for the treatment of an AIDS-related anemia, yet he insisted that he was in the early stages of illness. Although he claimed to see his condition as not very serious, he was also convinced that he would soon receive an early medical release. He focused all his attention on two inconsistent conditions: the possibility of early release by reason of a hopelessly terminal prognosis, and the hope of living until a cure could be discovered for AIDS.

Because early medical releases from prison are granted only to those with a terminal illness that is expected to lead to death in less than 6 months, or usually less then 3 months in actual practice, many prison patients face the same double-bind. Psychologically they need to deny the seriousness of the condition, yet they need simultaneously to acknowledge its seriousness in order to maintain hope for an early release.

Anger: Coping, Displacement, Inmate-Staff Hostility

As already noted, most prison inmates feel a great deal of anger and hostility regarding their incarceration but for those in the second stage of coping with dying, this anger borders on rage. Rando (1984) and Kubler-Ross (1969) discuss the appropriateness of the terminally ill patient's anger: it is both a way of coping with underlying feelings of grief, anxiety, and fear, and a perfectly normal reaction to the loss of control inherent in dying and in institutionalization. They stress that care givers need to be tolerant and understanding, allowing patients to express their anger within reasonable limits to avoid an unnecessary "escalation of aggressive behavior" (Rando, 1984, p.240) and to "help them toward a better acceptance of the final hours" (Kubler-Ross, 1969, p. 54).

Unfortunately, what often happens in the prison hospital, with its pervasive, almost inherent, distrust and tension between patients and staff is quite the opposite of what Rando and Kubler-Ross advocate. In the prison hospital there is an escalation of hostility and self-defeating, aggressive behavior. The patients tend to see the medical and correctional staff as the enemy. They use each other as convenient targets for displacement of anger. This ease with which prison inmates can project and displace their anger to staff may further delay the process of letting go of the anger and moving toward acceptance.

Case Example — Peter

Peter, a man in his early 50s with advanced liver and heart disease, was admitted to the hospice program with a prognosis of less than 3 months to live. He was convinced that his life could be saved or prolonged if he could just be released to care in an outside hospital. Peter believed his prison physician had given up on him, and he was intensely angry. He became extremely demanding and battled with the nurses and other staff including the inmate nursing attendants.

As a result people avoided him and he received a minimum of care. This, of course, made him even more angry. During one visit by a hospice volunteer, Peter flew into a rage. He leaped from his wheelchair and paced frantically back and forth. With tears streaming down his face, he agonized about the lack of care and attention he was receiving. Peter died a month later, angry and bitter to the end.

Bargaining and Hope:
Focus on Litigation and Early Release

Prison hospice patients bargain actively — in particular for early medical releases. They often participate in religious activities and pursue litigation. Although they may be resigned to their approaching death they want to taste freedom just one more time, or spend just a little time with their families again as free men. Very often they also hold to the hope theet once released they might obtain quality medical care and be cured.

The only chance of early release for most patients, however, is deterioration of their health to the point that death seems imminent. Thus, while patients bargain for more time and better health to pursue legal action for their release, any sign of actual improvement only diminishes the chance of early medical release. Patients often exhaust themselves in these efforts, becoming angry and bitterly resigned to dying in prison.

Case Example — John

John, a 55-year-old man with lung cancer, was admitted to the hospice program in deep depression shortly after having a court-ordered, early medical release overturned by the parole board because the prison medical staff reported he was responding to chemotherapy. As the initial depression lifted, John became energetic in litigating for his release. He worked to improve his health by eating more nutritiously and by being more physically active. He engaged in religious activities, cultivating a personal relationship with the visiting chaplain of his faith.

John's anger over the parole board's decision to cancel his previously granted early release never abated, however, and he remained obsessed with fighting that decision in the courts. He avoided any preparation for death and refused to deal with family conflicts that had arisen during his incarceration.

After about 6 months of this assertive activity, John gave up on his litigation efforts. He returned to a state of isolation and depression, became recalcitrant and exhibited bizarre behavior. He ate so little that a number of staff and prisoners who knew him well believed it was because he wanted his health to deteriorate so the parole board would release him. Staff insisted that the chemotherapy was working and that the cancer was in remission. John, on the other hand, insisted he was in constant pain and in fact dying.

Based on his rapidly deteriorating condition, the parole board did order John's release 2 months later. Although afraid he might die before reaching home, he was coherent and happy the day of the release. John died peacefully (according to the report of a friend) in a hospital near his home 3 days later.

As long as John held hope of release, he coped well with his fear of a lonely and shameful prison death, but when he relinquished that hope he became depressed and quickly deteriorated physically. Most prison patients, unlike John, never stop hoping that their situation will change or improve and they regularly express this hope until they enter the final physical stage of actually dying.

Prison hospice patients consistently express these two contradictory hopes: the hope for recovery and the hope for an early medical release from prison. The most often discussed issue and that of greatest concern to inmate hospice volunteers has been how to encourage patients to hope in general while helping them maintain some degree of realism about their situation in particular. As volunteers watch their patients and their patients' families ride the roller coaster of hope for cure and fear of dying in prison, they often become caught up in it themselves. Because such mood swings are exhausting, many prison hospice volunteers have become wary of becoming involved in this process at all. Nevertheless, this issue, unrealistic and futile as it may seem, is of primary concern to the majority of prisoner patients, and, therefore, must be addressed.

Depression: Pathological and Functional States

When the inevitability of dying in prison becomes obvious to a patient, hopelessness, despair, and deep depression often follow. This depression may be situational—brought on by a combination of incarceration, illness, and loss of hope. Or it may be functional—the "preparatory depression" (Kubler-Ross, 1969, p. 86) that normally occurs in the latter stages of the dying process.

In the first case, the premature onset of depression often reaches pathological proportions in the prison setting, actually accelerating the dying process. The stigma and sense of failure associated with dying in prison, the fear of dying alone, and the depressing environment all contribute to episodes of despair and sometimes suicidal behavior. Because hospice patients are frequently in this state of reactive and potentially pathological depression when referred to the program, the program volunteers generally try to engage them as soon as possible in any kind of positive activity that returns some meaning and hope to their lives.

That this depression has quickly lifted in some cases, as some of the patients' basic psychosocial needs begin to be met with the help of their volunteers, has been one of the more obvious successes of the program. In fact, in some cases patients who were considered near death at the time of referral to the program have made what seem to be dramatic physical recoveries, often to the point that they want to see a volunteer only to keep the relationship alive in case of a change.

In most cases, however, the elation seen at this stage is temporary, and at some point as the dying process progresses the hospice volunteer must consciously shift his attention to the patient's need to prepare for death.

As they make this shift, the volunteers find they need to deal with their own anticipatory grief at losing this person in whom they have invested so much caring and who may have become a close friend. Indeed, because the hospice volunteers in the prison setting often become the sole emotional and psychological support for their patients, especially in the later stages of the dying process, inmate volunteers may become surrogate family members. Thus for them the patient's death results in deep bereavement and grieving.

Case Example — Roger

A 37-year-old man named Roger was admitted to the hospice program with advanced AIDS. The hospice volunteer found Roger in a state of complete despair and isolation. On "lock-down" status, he had lost his TV because of an angry outburst at a guard in which he had thrown his meal tray to the floor. He was unshaven; his hair was long, unwashed, and uncombed; his overall hygiene was poor; and his room disordered and dirty. Roger had simply stopped caring for himself.

After several weeks of companionship, attention, and encouragement from his volunteer, however, Roger made a complete turnaround: he cut his hair, began to shave again, and became fastidious about his hygiene and the cleanliness of his room. He also began attending religious services with his volunteer, and gained a new hope for extending his life and possibly returning home.

Case Example — Tyler

At the time of his referral to the hospice program Tyler, a 50-year-old man dying of AIDS, was very hopeful of receiving an early release. He talked freely with his volunteer, and gradually they established a strong relationship. They attended leisure activities and religious services together and sometimes prayed together in Tyler's room. Suddenly Tyler lost interest and vitality, became withdrawn, depressed, and uncommunicative to the point of often falling asleep during visits from his volunteer. He began refusing food, became agitated and paced the halls at night.

The volunteer at first felt that something—possibly in relation to his family—had occurred in Tyler's life and that he wasn't sharing it. The volunteer questioned Tyler about it. Tyler said that nothing had happened and that there was nothing he really needed to talk about. He assured his volunteer that he was still at peace with God and himself. He continued to withdraw physically and emotionally, and within a few weeks he died. By that time, the volunteer had come to realize that Tyler was simply withdrawing from the relationship as he prepared for death.

Final Stages: Acceptance or Realization of the Inevitable—Trusting the Dying Process

The acceptance stage described by Kubler-Ross (1969) as the last stage of dying may actually occur infrequently in the general population (Humphrey, cited in Rando, 1984). In our experience it is infrequent among prison hospice patients, as well. The psychological and spiritual work involved in reaching any degree of acceptance is made all the more difficult by the fear and shame these patients feel in anticipation of a lonely prison death. Prisoners simply cannot experience the "appropriate death" defined by Weisman as "one that a person might choose, had he a choice" (cited in Buschman, 1986, p. 84). Most feel only bitter resignation at their situation. For this reason, it may be unrealistic to make facilitating the acceptance of death a primary goal of inmate volunteers' psychosocial interventions with their patients.

Humphrey notes that in the general population what occurs more often than acceptance of death is a "realization of the inevitable" (Rando, 1984, p. 268). In other words, though the patient may never be at peace with death or the losses it entails, he or she can, at least, move beyond denial into acknowledging the reality of approaching death. This sense of realism about the inevitability of death that prison patients can feel is perhaps a more practical goal of psychosocial intervention.

An even more reasonable approach to working with dying prisoners may be to allow them to experience the dying process naturally, avoiding a goal orientation altogether. Ostaseski suggests as much in discussing his work as director of a San Francisco hospice program: "I've never had a situation in which I couldn't trust the dying process. It's very potent; it does its own work, just like the birth process does" (quoted in Addonizio, 1989, p. 5). Humphrey (cited in Rando, 1984) also makes this analogy between the final stage of death and the birth process. Inmate hospice volunteers have often seen in the latter stages of their patients' dying process this withdrawal and absorption into the moment. The patient's anger, shame, and bitterness about dying in prison become irrelevant as death actually begins to occur and the patient appears to have "one foot in another world" (Rando, 1984, p. 269). The patient's greatest concern often becomes simply not to be left alone.

CONCLUSION AND RECOMMENDATIONS

In this examination of the sociocultural world and psychosocial experiences and needs of terminally ill and dying prisoners, it is apparent that these individuals are in a unique situation: they have many added tasks to work through to attain any semblance of a good death — or at least a death that is not filled with anger, bitterness, and despair — in prison.

Most of the issues discussed in this paper have been addressed by Rando (1984), Buschman (1986), Zimmerman (1986), and others in relation to a variety of medical care environments. In the correctional setting these same issues take on added dimension and intensity. This situation should be formally researched if we are to develop a better understanding of the needs of prisoners and the best ways to meet those needs.

The inmate-staffed hospice volunteer program from which the information in this article comes was developed by concerned inmates and prison staff in what may have been the first concerted effort to use the hospice model to address the needs of patients dying in a correctional setting. A similar program has now been started at another federal prison medical facility in Rochester, Minnesota, and administrators at California's primary correctional medical facility at Vacaville are considering developing a palliative care program there, as well. With the rapid growth and steady aging of prison populations throughout the country, it is hoped that administrators in the other 49 state correctional systems are now or will soon be considering taking an organized approach to palliative medical care for dying prisoners.

Present efforts need to be broadened to include full-service hospice care for dying prisoners and their families or significant others. This service should include the use of inmate volunteers, volunteer staff support, an interdisciplinary approach with hospice protocols for pain management, accommodation for extensive family visitation, and provision of bereavement services to family, friends, and staff.

To meet these goals, consideration should be given to developing free-standing palliative care units for prisoners. Such units could provide the same services as do current community hospice programs, while still meeting the security needs of the institution. Such units could provide a safe environment in which patients, their families, and their caregivers could attend to the final stage of life with dignity and compassion.

REFERENCES

Addonizio, K. (August, 1989). Living with death and dying, an interview with Frank Ostaseski. *The Sun*. San Francisco, CA, 165, 2-4.

Buschman, M. (1986). Psychosocial issues in the care of the terminally ill. In J. M. Zimmerman (Ed.), *Hospice, complete care for the terminally ill* (2nd ed.) (pp. 77-90). Baltimore-Munich: Urban & Schwarzenberg.

Heffernan, E. (1972). *Making it in prison*. New York: John Wiley & Sons.

Kelly, P. (1988). Kubler-Ross's stages of death model applied to Darkness at Noon. *Criminal Justice and Behavior*, 21, 172-178.

Kubler-Ross, E. (1969). *On death and dying*. New York: Collier/Macmillan.

Kubler-Ross, E. (1987). *AIDS: The ultimate challenge*. New York: Collier/Macmillan.

Lacayo, R. (1989, May 29). Our bulging prisons. *Time*, pp. 28-31.

National Institute of Justice/Issues Practices. 1989 Update: AIDS in correctional facilities. (May, 1990). Washington DC: United States Department of Justice.

Rando, T. (1984). *Grief, dying, and death: Clinical interventions for care givers*. Champagne, IL: Research Press.

Zimmerman, J. (1986). *Hospice, complete care for the terminally ill* (2nd ed.). Baltimore-Munich: Urban and Schwarzenberg.

Grieving a Loss from AIDS

J. William Worden

SUMMARY. The determinants of the nature of an AIDS death and their likely effects on the survivors are identified. Specifically discussed with illustrative case examples are stigma, lack of social support, contagion, untimely death, protracted illness and disfigurement, and neurological complications. Strategies for intervention are suggested.

INTRODUCTION

Since 1981 an ever increasing number of people have become afflicted with and died from Acquired Immune Deficiency Syndrome (AIDS). It is estimated by the year 2000 a half-million people in the United States will have died from AIDS-related disorders. Each of those who die will leave family and friends to face the consequences particular to this type of loss. Survivors of those who die from AIDS constitute a population of mourners with few existing guidelines for care (Oerlemans-Bunn, 1988).

Any person's grief response is influenced by a series of determinants that affect both the intensity and course of the mourning (Worden, 1985). Such determinants include the relationship to the deceased, the nature of the attachment, the person's history of losses, and social support. An important determinant is the type of death that took the deceased. Sudden deaths are grieved differently

J. William Worden, PhD, is Professor of Psychology at the Rosemead School of Psychology (California) and Principal Investigator of the Child Bereavement Study at the Harvard Medical School/Massachusetts General Hospital. He is also Psychological Consultant to the AIDS research project at Columbia University and to the Hospice of Pasadena, CA.

Address correspondence to the author c/o Child Bereavement Study, Department of Psychiatry, Massachusetts General Hospital, Boston, MA 02114.

than expected deaths. Deaths that are natural as the consequence of disease are grieved differently than traumatic deaths.

There are several features of an AIDS death that can have bearing on a survivor's reaction. That the syndrome is caused by an infectious virus, currently lacks a cure, carries a social stigma, and often leads to protracted illness all influence the mourning behavior of the survivors. In this paper I present several of the salient features of an AIDS death that can influence grieving behavior in order to help counselors improve the effectiveness of their interventions.

STIGMA

There are certain deaths that result in socially unspeakable losses, i.e., people find it difficult to talk about them. There is often a conscious conspiracy of silence that develops around the loss (Worden, 1991). One example is death by suicide. AIDS is another. An AIDS death tends to carry a stigma whether the victim is homosexual, heterosexual, an IV drug user, a child infected through transfusion, or an infant infected in utero.

Because of this stigma, some survivors fear they will be rejected and judged harshly if the cause of the death becomes known. Persons may lie and attribute the death to cancer or some cause other than AIDS. Although this may temporarily get them off the "AIDS hook," such deception in the long run takes its emotional toll in fear of discovery, anger that a cover-up seems necessary, and possible guilt over what they have done.

Case Example

Harold and Mary live in a small midwest town and their only son Michael died of AIDS in San Francisco. They had never been sure of their son's lifestyle and his death as a result of the HIV virus distressed them. Neither of them felt they could share the cause of death with others so they made up the story that he had died in an automobile accident. Several months later they felt so contrite about this lie that they shared the truth with their church congregation. Rather than being rejected and judged they found support and love.

Their disclosure also helped two other couples in the church share their privately held concerns about their own children's sexuality.

Counselors can help survivors to deal with this perceived stigma and to test the reality of what might happen if others found out or knew the real cause of death. Counselors can also assist survivors to find appropriate persons and more comfortable ways to share the circumstances of the loss. Role playing such interactions can be a useful intervention.

Elsewhere I have identified four tasks of mourning that one must accomplish when accommodating to a loss (Worden, 1982). The first task of mourning — accepting the reality of the loss — can be facilitated by talking about the loss including its circumstances. If an AIDS survivor has difficulty doing this, the counselor can be an important person to actively listen, to hear the story told over and over again until the person begins to accept its reality. This, together with encouragement to share this information with others, can do much to help attenuate feelings of anxiety and fear that go along with such stigma.

Persons like Ryan White and the family of Paul Michael Glaser who go public with their AIDS problem may help to counter the AIDS stigma. However, as long as the AIDS epidemic continues to place serious strains on our economic and health care resources it will probably continue to be seen as a stigmatized type of death, particularly by those who see it as preventable.

LACK OF SOCIAL SUPPORT

Kinship in our society legitimizes grief. Many survivors who have had a nontraditional relationship with the deceased have difficulty finding the level of understanding and support they need from others after the death. The mother of one client, who did not know of her son's relationship with his lover, said to him after the death, "Why are you so sad? He was only your roommate." If a relationship is not socially sanctioned, it is less likely to be recognized as important by others or by the law. There have been several instances where the family may exclude the deceased's partners and friends from participation in funeral planning and activities. Significant others in the deceased's life may be prevented from inheriting property or otherwise benefitting from the settlement of the estate.

Folta and Deck make an important point about grief and nontraditional relationships: "While all of these studies tell us that grief is a normal phenomenon, the intensity of which corresponds to the closeness of the relationship with the deceased, they fail to take friendship into account. The underlying assumption is that 'closeness of relationship' exists only among spouses and or immediate kin" (Folta & Deck, 1976, p. 239).

Groups established for families and friends of AIDS patients can be excellent means of providing emotional support before and after the death. Counselors can help in setting up such groups and providing leadership for them.

CONTAGION

Because AIDS is a sexually transmitted disease, the sexual partners of the deceased may be anxious about their own health. Physical symptoms usually considered a normal part of the grieving process such as fatigue, insomnia, and headaches can be interpreted by partners as symptoms associated with AIDS-related illnesses (Martin, 1988). Counselors need to educate survivors about these physical aspects of normal bereavement so that those symptoms are not construed as AIDS. Doing so may cause the anxiety stemming from these physical symptoms to abate.

Physical symptoms can also be overt manifestations of suppressed guilt. If this is the case, then the counselor can help the person to identify the guilt, help him or her test it in relation to reality, and if real culpability exists, to find appropriate ways of working through the guilt to find self-forgiveness and peace of mind.

On the other hand, a counselor should never presume that physical symptoms the bereaved complain of are psychological in origin. Advising clients to get appropriate medical check-ups and clinical testing is always in order. If a medical evaluation proves negative, the counselor can then facilitate the working through of any underlying psychological conflicts.

Some survivors may feel guilty for transmitting the virus to their partner or for participating in activities or in a lifestyle in which the possibility of transmission was heightened. These feelings of guilt need to be evaluated and worked through.

Contagion factors can also play a role when a survivor starts to establish new relationships. Some people reject close relationships with AIDS survivors.

Case Example

Dean had recently lost his companion of 6 years to AIDS. After a sufficient period of mourning he decided to reenter the social scene and move on with his life. Even though he was not HIV positive, he was surprised to find that most of the people he met socially, once they knew about his previous relationship, shied away from any serious involvement with him.

In other cases the survivors themselves may have doubts about forming new relationships. The counselor can help persons to deal with their feelings regarding either of these situations. Of particular importance are the identification of cognitive messages and self-talk that survivors may be giving themselves such as, "No one will ever love me again." Identifying these thought patterns, beliefs, and assumptions and working with them are important counseling goals in order to attenuate feelings of depression and anxiety that often accompany distorted cognition (Beck, 1967).

UNTIMELY DEATHS

Many of those who have succumbed to an AIDS-related illness are young, a large number between the ages of 20 and 35. Their deaths elicit the same reactions that any untimely death can provoke (Weisman, 1973).

Among the friends and contemporaries of these young victims there can be an increased awareness of personal mortality with its attendant anxiety (Worden, 1976). For most of us our personal death awareness exists at a low level of consciousness moving to the forefront when we have a close brush with death ourselves, lose the last of our parents, or lose a contemporary to death. "He was much too young to die," said a friend of his 29 year old housemate.

Implicit in this comment was the statement, "I am too young to die. This cannot happen to me yet." Existential anxiety is an expected correlate of increased personal death awareness and each of us copes with this anxiety through long established personal coping patterns—some more effective than others. The counselor working with bereaved AIDS survivors needs to be alert to existential anxiety and other feelings associated with personal death awareness and to help the client deal with this in as direct and healthy a manner as possible.

Loss of a child is counted among the most serious. Children are supposed to outlive their parents. Bereaved parents losing children from any type of death have a difficult adjustment. The addition of the stigma of an AIDS death compounds it. I have worked with several parents who did not know the lifestyle of their child until after the death. For them, they not only had to grieve the youth whom they lost to death, they also had to grieve the child they thought they had and did not, as part of their overall bereavement.

PROTRACTED ILLNESS AND DISFIGUREMENT

Many of the opportunistic infections characteristic of AIDS can and do lead to progressive physical and mental deterioration. Persons with AIDS become wasted physically and mentally. Formerly youthful and attractive, they are transformed into the likenesses of death camp victims. When this type of deterioration occurs there are those who find it difficult to be around persons with AIDS. They tell themselves, "I prefer to remember him as he was." After the death, however, some who have taken this remote posture feel strong guilt because they were not there when the person was dying. If this guilt is sufficient to bring them for counseling, the counselor can help them try to deal with it. Active techniques such as letter writing, using the Gestalt empty chair, or grief work done at the gravesite can often facilitate the working through of such guilt.

Others who have not abandoned the person who was dying and were present through the dying process may find it difficult to relinquish memories of a friend or family member in such an impaired condition. A counselor can help the survivor realize that this is normal and that gradually over time they will be able to recapture a more balanced set of memories.

Case Example

Bob was a handsome model with a gregarious personality. As the ravages of AIDS progressed he took on the appearance of a frail-elderly old man. People who had not seen him for awhile, but saw him toward the end of his life, were shocked by this change in appearance. Some of his friends stayed away when they heard how much he had changed. Others came to be with him during his final days. What was helpful for many of them was to have an earlier photograph of Bob present at the memorial service so they could remember him as he had been and not just as he looked toward the end of his life.

NEUROLOGICAL COMPLICATIONS

Another feature of AIDS that impacts loss are the frequently severe neurological complications. Sometimes the damage makes for subtle changes in behavior but more often one sees a more gross level of impairment depending on the area of the brain that is under attack by the virus. These deteriorations of mental function can often mimic the impairments suffered in Alzheimer's disease.

Once the dementia progresses, family and friends begin to feel the loss of the person they once loved, and these losses may precipitate early grieving. Although some grieving can be done in anticipation of the death, additional grieving must be done following the death when the final reality of the loss sets in. Counselors who work with patients and their loved ones can provide an understanding of this process and work with them to maintain an appropriate contact that will help maintain the patient's quality of life before the death and the survivors' bereavement after the loss.

CONCLUSION

The AIDS virus continues to infect a broader segment of the population and will probably continue to affect a larger portion of society than we have seen to date. No longer is the syndrome limited to 2 or 3 specific target groups. It is no longer a gay disease or one restricted to IV drug use. One of the alarming conditions is the spread of the virus among women, infants, and the young heterosexual segment of our society. Counselors need to stay abreast of these demographic changes and be prepared to offer assistance to those seeking help both before the death and afterwards.

REFERENCES

Beck, A. T. (1976). *Cognitive therapy and the emotional disorders*. New York: International Universities Press.

Folta, J. & E. Deck. (1986). Grief, the funeral, and the friend, in V. Pine et al. (Eds). *Acute grief and the funeral*. Springfield, IL: Thomas.

Martin, J. L. (1988). Psychological consequences of AIDS- related bereavement among gay men. *Journal of Clinical & Consulting Psychology*, 56, 856-862.

Oerlemans-Bunn, M. (1988). On being gay, single, and bereaved. *American Journal of Nursing*, 88, 472-476.

Worden, J. W. (1985). Bereavement. *Seminars in Oncology* 12, 472-475.

Worden, J. W. (1976). *Personal death awareness*. Englewood Cliffs, NJ: Prentice-Hall.

Worden, J. W. (1982). *Grief counseling and grief therapy: A handbook for the mental health practitioner*. New York: Springer.

Worden, J.W. (in press). *Grief counseling and grief therapy: A handbook for the mental health practitioner*. (2nd ed.) New York: Springer.

AIDS in the Workplace:
Implications for Hospice Programs

Dorothy N. Moga
Sharon E. Brodeur
Peggy Beckman

SUMMARY. AIDS presents health care providers with complex medical management issues as well as the need to confront their own fears and prejudices. Hospice programs provide specialized care to persons who are in the final stages of the disease. As the epidemic grows, they increasingly also must respond to HIV-infected staff. A comprehensive workplace program prepares the hospice provider for these challenges and ensures an appropriate response. The four essential elements of such a program are policy development, staff education, supervisory training, and compliance monitoring. Policies to consider include infection control, occupational exposure, confidentiality, and the response to HIV-infected patients and employees. Comprehensive education ensures quality care for AIDS patients. Particularly crucial is the education of managers and supervisors. After policy implementation and training, procedures must

Dorothy N. Moga, MPH, is Assistant Vice President, Fairfax Hospital System, Inova Health Systems; Co-chair, Inova AIDS Task Force; member of several community boards, including Hospice of Northern Virginia; member, National Hospice Organization AIDS Resource Committee; and was Administrator, Hospice of Northern Virginia, 1979-1986. Sharon E. Brodeur, BSN, MPA, is Director of HIV Services, Inova Health Systems; member, Metropolitan Washington Regional HIV Health Services Planning Council; and President, Board of Directors, Northern Virginia AIDS Ministry. Peggy Beckman, BSN, is Coordinator of Clinical Services, Office of HIV Services, Inova Health Systems; a consultant and trainer on AIDS in the workplace and AIDS patient care; and co-leader of a support group for mothers of HIV-infected persons.

The authors would like to thank Delia Mason for her editing of the manuscript.

Address correspondence to Dorothy N. Moga, Fairfax Hospital System, 8001 Braddock Road, Springfield, VA 22151.

be instituted to monitor compliance and develop corrective action. A bibliography of additional resource materials is provided.

INTRODUCTION

At present patients with AIDS have an average life expectancy of 18 months from the time of diagnosis. During the final stages of the disease hospice programs can provide them the appropriate level of needed care. Although care of an AIDS patient at home may present almost overwhelming challenges to family and/or friends, a well-prepared hospice program can provide the required support just as such programs have facilitated home care for patients with other terminal illnesses. Increasingly patients and their families, physicians, and community service providers are recognizing the important role of hospice, and especially home care services in the continuum of care. As the number of people with AIDS increases, the demand for hospice care for them will grow.

The AIDS epidemic calls for all health care providers to adhere strictly to universal precautions and infection control techniques, to keep abreast of rapidly breaking medical advances, and to confront their own personal stereotypic thinking and prejudices. Hospice workers who care for patients with AIDS may need to cope with patients the same age as themselves or their children, and with patients lacking the social, psychological, and economic support systems usually available to other patients. Another challenge confronted by health care and hospice programs is dealing with staff — "staff" is used throughout to refer to both employees and volunteers — who may be infected with HIV. To meet this challenge, the employer must help staff to adjust relationships with other employees and with volunteers, to interpret benefit packages, and to decide on the degree of flexibility in work assignments. Caring for patients with AIDS or discovering that a staff member is HIV-infected can create disruption and confusion, but such a response can be avoided by the development of comprehensive policies and programs for staff education. This article helps prepare the hospice program to respond to either the patient or the staff member with HIV infection or AIDS.

The four elements essential to a comprehensive workplace program are policy development, staff education, supervisory training, and compliance monitoring.

POLICY DEVELOPMENT

Comprehensive policies are the framework within which a program provides effective care for patients with AIDS or responds appropriately to HIV infection in a staff member. Staff may initially be anxious when expected to care for or work with a person with AIDS. They may fear accidental transmission of HIV, or they may be reluctant to care for someone who is gay or bisexual or an IV drug user. Some agencies have had high staff turnover after admitting an AIDS patient. However, when these concerns are anticipated and openly addressed and sound policies are coupled with appropriate education, such responses can be attenuated if not outright prevented.

Policy development is also essential in protecting the program from litigation. Agencies must meet local, state, and federal legislative requirements and regulations that govern hiring practices as well as the care of persons with AIDS.

The landmark civil rights legislation of the decade, the Americans with Disabilities Act, enacted in August 1990, protects disabled people, including those who are or who are perceived to be HIV-infected, by prohibiting employers from engaging in any form of discriminatory behavior. For example, an employee cannot be asked to undergo HIV testing unless all employees are tested. The law also requires that persons who are disabled be accommodated in the workplace. This includes permitting them to work flexible hours, providing them time off for medical appointments, and altering facilities to ensure access to them. State laws that may have an impact on program policies include those that mandate testing a patient for HIV if a staff member is exposed to the patient's blood or body fluids or reporting the names of HIV-infected persons to the state health department.

Regulations of particular importance for all employers are the Occupational Safety and Health Administration proposed rule on bloodborne pathogens (OSHA, 1989) and the CDC guidelines on universal precautions, infection control, and HIV exposure (CDC,

1989). OSHA is already authorized to inspect and issue citations to health care facilities based on section 5A1 of the existing standards—the "general duty" clause—which requires employers to provide a safe workplace for employees. OSHA specifically expects compliance with CDC guidelines on personal protective equipment, hazardous waste disposal, infection control, and universal precautions.

Forming a Strategy Team

Forming a strategy team is the first step in determining which policies are needed, who develops and reviews them, and how they are to be implemented. The ideal team should include representatives from senior management, human resources, and nursing—both home care and inpatient—and a physician with expertise in infectious diseases to provide input during policy development and review. The number of people may be limited in small programs, but the team should always seek input from those in the disciplines listed, even if only on a consultant basis.

Assessing Policies To Be Developed

The first task for the strategy team is to assess the organization's need for policies. Although the team will want to consider all six of the following policies, the first two are essential.

Universal precautions and infection control policy. The universal precautions and infection control policy should be based on the most current CDC guidelines and OSHA regulations. In addition, policies developed for inpatient settings must meet local requirements for handling infectious waste. For all settings this policy should include a section identifying potentially infectious body fluids, and it should provide explicit information on the use of barrier precautions. It should address homecare-specific concerns; e.g., protection of the patient from infection, proper techniques for handling laundry, kitchen activities, maintenance of bathrooms, waste disposal, needles and other sharps disposal, creation of a disinfectant solution, cleanup of blood and other body fluids, and sharing of personal items such as toothbrushes or razors. Special attention should be paid to the appropriate use of gowns, gloves, masks, and eye shields.

HIV/Hepatitis B exposure and vaccination policy. Although the risk of HIV infection from an occupational exposure is small (0.47%) (Marcus et al., 1988; CDC, 1989), the lack of a cure for HIV infection makes the risk of exposure a critical concern. Because the risk of hepatitis B (HBV) seroconversion after one needlestick is 12% to 17% (CDC, 1987b), exposure to HBV, which is transmitted similarly to HIV, is also a serious concern. Policies for managing exposure of health personnel to these organisms need to address the program's response after an exposure and they must ensure that every possible precaution is taken to protect the staff person's health. Because the procedures for handling HIV and HBV exposures are different, it may be advisable to write two policies. Each policy should include provisions for testing the patient who was the source of the exposure when the patient's HIV or HBV status is unknown and, if the patient tests positive, for testing the exposed staff member.

The CDC recommends that when the patient is HIV-positive the exposed staff member be retested at 6 weeks, at 12 weeks, and at 6 months. Testing must be accompanied by appropriate counseling, teaching, and recommendations for preventing transmission, to be used until follow-up is complete (CDC, 1987a).

If the patient is positive for HBV, the staff person should be tested for antibodies and, if they are not present, he or she should receive both the HBV vaccine and immunoglobulin (CDC, 1987b). Given the risk of conversion after an occupational exposure to HBV, vaccination of all staff who are at risk of exposure should be seriously considered and will be mandated by the new OSHA regulations. Vaccines currently available carry a low risk of side effects.

Confidentiality policy. Confidentiality is particularly important if a patient is infected with HIV. The number of staff who know the diagnosis should be limited to those who care for him or her. Widespread discussion of the diagnosis or the placement of blood and body fluid precaution signs outside a patient's room are not necessary for safe care. Because they arouse suspicion about the patient's HIV status they should be avoided. If the staff person tests positive for HIV, he or she must be assured that such information will be kept confidential. Such assurance complies with regulations requiring confidentiality of employee medical records and it also enables the worker to discuss his or her HIV positivity more openly with supervisors.

Personnel policy on HIV-infected employees. The management of the hospice program may question the need for special personnel policies governing its response to HIV-infected workers when it already has chronic or life-threatening illness policies in place. Such policies are needed because AIDS is still so associated with fear, discrimination, and misunderstanding that it is advantageous for the hospice program to have a separate policy.

The personnel policy should include information about disability leave (with or without pay), medical insurance continuation, use of accrued vacation and sick time, and use of personal time for health-related appointments. Perhaps even more difficult to resolve is whether HIV-infected employees and volunteers will be permitted to continue to provide patient care. The personnel policy should provide guidelines for the management of all these issues.

Personnel policy on care of HIV-infected patients. Will the hospice program permit staff to refuse to care for AIDS patients? Before a patient with AIDS is admitted to a hospice inpatient facility or to a hospice home care program, the organization's position on this issue should be clear. Internal discussion may reveal differing viewpoints, but the program's position on staff responsibilities, once determined, must be supported by senior management and the governing body. This is an issue that can be complicated if the program uses non-hospice personnel to supplement care in the home, or if the hospice program does not control which cases are accepted by other agency staff. The hospice program may want to consider developing a special pool of workers committed to providing care to patients with AIDS.

Internal and External Resources
to Assist Policy Development

The next step in developing policies is to identify internal and external resources to help in the process. The CDC guidelines (CDC, 1987a) and update (CDC, 1988) on universal precautions are invaluable in developing policies on universal precautions, HIV exposure, and infection control. The OSHA proposed rule (OSHA, 1990) provides guidelines for developing policies and procedures for HBV and HIV exposures and requirements regarding HBV vaccination. An infection control practitioner can assist in resolving such practical questions as, "How do you dispose of soiled dressings in the home?" If the hospice does not have a nurse with infection control expertise on staff, it might consider a consultant arrangement with an infection control practitioner from a local hospital or home care agency.

Educating and Gaining the Support of the Governing Board and Senior Management

It is important to engage senior management in discussions early in the course of policy development. Senior management and the board of directors must agree that the goal of HIV policy development and educational programs is to prepare staff to care effectively and compassionately for patients with AIDS and their families and to ensure the safety of all employees. There must also be consensus, consistent with legislative requirements and the facts about HIV, in the development of an organizational response to HIV-infected staff. Since board members rely on senior management for much of their information, it is critical that senior managers agree with the need for such policies and that they understand the regulatory environment in which they have been drafted. Without senior management and board understanding, support for implementation will be difficult.

The successful organization and implementation of policy development and training is dependent on an extensive commitment of staff time and energy. Without senior management leadership and support, it would be difficult for a hospice program to commit the resources required to develop and implement necessary policies.

Implementation of Policies

The implementation of universal precautions and infection control policies has a budgetary impact in that personal protective equipment must be purchased. This equipment includes gloves, gowns, masks, eye wear, sharps containers, and disinfectant solutions. Supplies have to be stocked, and home care staff, PRN pool staff, and inpatient staff, including housekeeping, need to be trained in their use. Exposure policies influence the maintenance of staff health records and call for new employee health procedures such as obtaining consent for and performing the tests for HIV and HBV. Prior to actual implementation of policies, all such considerations need to be addressed. The supplies should be on hand and readily accessible and the personnel must be oriented to their use.

Slightly different strategies will be required to implement each policy. Therefore, policy development also includes analyzing implementation tasks, assigning work, and establishing the time frames for implementation.

STAFF EDUCATION

AIDS presents caregivers with complex problems and symptoms that are difficult to control. A comprehensive education program is essential to ensure high-quality, compassionate care for the HIV-infected patient and his or her family and to allow staff to be comfortable and confident in their ability to provide that care. Ideally, education takes place prior to the admission of the first HIV-infected patient or the discovery of an infected staff member. Education should help staff recognize and modify their negative feelings about individuals who are HIV-infected. It should also provide them with the information they need to care effectively for patients with AIDS while ensuring that their own risk for occupational exposure is low. Because AIDS is a newly recognized disease and treatment methods change rapidly, it is important that staff stay current.

An agency's approach to developing an educational program will vary depending on size. Ideally, human resources staff will assist in educating workers about personnel policies. If the program is small, the executive director or whoever handles personnel matters may conduct the training. Orienting and training staff in infection control and universal precautions procedures should be performed by an infection control nurse or a nurse who is well versed in infection control practices. Staff should be allowed time to ask questions and raise concerns.

The person selected to conduct HIV-related training must know how to treat HIV-infected patients and must be committed to ongoing education in this area. The trainer must be comfortable with eliciting feelings from staff, nonjudgmental, and able to help staff resolve their concerns by listening and providing accurate information. It may be useful to recruit a consultant to assist the designated staff person in developing and implementing the first training module. The staff person can then continue as the inhouse trainer.

Needs Assessment

The trainer will find it helpful to perform a formal needs assessment to elicit staff concerns and to evaluate the level of knowledge about HIV (see Figure 1 for a sample needs assessment). The training program should be designed based on OSHA requirements, established program policies, and the results of the needs assessment. The program should be offered to all levels of staff, to management, to volunteers, and to families of patients. OSHA currently requires training in the language of and at the literacy level of the learner (OSHA, 1990). If English is a second language for one or more staff members, the trainer will have to find a translator. The organization may be able to enlist employees or volunteers from other appropriate community-based organizations.

Education/Training Plan

The needs assessment will identify areas for concentration with specific groups of learners, but basic information must first be presented to ensure that everyone starts with the same knowledge base. For example, a unique aspect of AIDS is the element of fear and prejudice associated with it. Most caregivers have not experienced working with people with a disease that simultaneously is infectious and terminal, and involves large numbers of people from deviant social groups viewed with prejudice and discrimination. AIDS raises all these issues, and the strong feelings that accompany them need to be addressed before information about caring for patients with AIDS can be taken in.

An excellent setting in which to address these matters is the staff support group, a feature of most hospice programs. If such support

FIGURE 1

Northern Virginia HIV Resource and Consultation Center
Needs Assessment Part I
HIV Infection and AIDS

1. What is your position?

   ☐ RN   ☐ LPN   ☐ Nursing Assistant   ☐ Volunteer

   ☐ Other Caregiving   ☐ Other Non-Caregiving

2. Have you had direct caregiving experience with AIDS patients?

   _____

3. What are your major concerns in providing care?

   _____
   _____
   _____

4. What educational meetings have you attended, either here or outside, on the subject of HIV infection?

   _____
   _____
   _____

5. Please rate the following education topics in terms of importance for you.

	Very Important	Important	Not at all Important		
a. Basic information about HIV infection	5	4	3	2	1
b. Ways to prevent infection	5	4	3	2	1
c. Nursing care and symptom management	5	4	3	2	1
d. Medications/treatments	5	4	3	2	1
e. Knowledge about homosexuality	5	4	3	2	1
f. Sexuality	5	4	3	2	1
g. Safer sex	5	4	3	2	1
h. Substance abuse	5	4	3	2	1
i. Women and HIV infection	5	4	3	2	1
j. Opportunistic infections	5	4	3	2	1
k. Psychosocial needs of the patient	5	4	3	2	1
l. Psychosocial needs of the family	5	4	3	2	1
m. Support for professional caregiving staff	5	4	3	2	1
n. Legal/ethical issues	5	4	3	2	1
o. Clinical research update	5	4	3	2	1
p. Neuropsychological manifestations	5	4	3	2	1
q. Community research update	5	4	3	2	1
r. Other	5	4	3	2	1

_____
_____

groups do not meet on a regular basis, time should be allotted for personal awareness groups limited to 12 workers. At these meetings staff can talk about their experiences, attitudes, and feelings. The objectives are to identify fears and feelings that hinder the caregiver in establishing a therapeutic relationship with the patient and fam-

Northern Virginia HIV Resource and Consultation Center
Needs Assessment Part II
HIV Infection and AIDS

Please circle the response which best describes your feelings about working with patients with HIV infection and AIDS. Please take a minute to think about the statement. There are no right or wrong answers (3 = Strongly agree; 2 = agree; 1 = strongly disagree).

1. I feel I don't know enough about the disease to be able to provide good care.   3 2 1
2. I am worried about taking the disease home to my family.   3 2 1
3. I feel comfortable providing care to someone who is an IV drug abuser.   3 2 1
4. I can provide good care to the family and significant others of AIDS patients.   3 2 1
5. I feel uncomfortable with most homosexual behavior.   3 2 1
6. I share no values or beliefs with most gay people.   3 2 1
7. I am concerned about getting AIDS.   3 2 1
8. I feel this group of patients represents a professional challenge.   3 2 1
9. I feel more compassion for hemophiliacs and infants with AIDS than for those who acquire AIDS through sex or IV routes.   3 2 1
10. I feel homosexuals represent a broad range of behavior, values, and attitudes. I have some things in common with some homosexuals.   3 2 1
11. I feel angry about women giving AIDS to their babies.   3 2 1
12. I feel comfortable in my knowledge of the addictive process and my ability to handle the addicted patient.   3 2 1
13. I feel angry with men who have infected their female partners.   3 2 1
14. I don't approve of a homosexual lifestyle, but feel I can provide good care to the gay AIDS patient.   3 2 1
15. I feel uncomfortable around homosexuals who are openly affectionate with each other.   3 2 1
16. I find the substance-abusing patient very difficult to manage.   3 2 1
17. My family is very frightened of my work with AIDS patients.   3 2 1
18. I find it difficult to work with young patients who are dying.   3 2 1
19. I cannot talk about my work with AIDS patients with my family.   3 2 1
20. I think staff should have the choice not to work with AIDS patients.   3 2 1
21. I feel I am always consistent with universal precautions.   3 2 1
22. I worry about other staff members' use of precautions.   3 2 1
23. I tend to consider the circumstances rather than explicitly following agency policies.   3 2 1

ily, to explore these feelings, and to establish a process for resolving such concerns.

A professional facilitator experienced in the care of AIDS patients and in the use of role play or interactive exercises can stimulate discussion. One very effective strategy for stimulating discussion and reducing fear is to ask a person with AIDS to speak about his or her experience of living with the condition. Or, the facilitator might show any of a number of excellent films on this topic. At least 30 minutes should be allotted for participants to ask questions of the guest speaker or to discuss the film.

After participants' feelings have been addressed, the basic facts about HIV infection should be presented to all levels of staff — administrative, support, maintenance, volunteer, and clinical. The following topics should be included: epidemiology; transmission; the continuum of HIV infection; testing; symptoms, diagnosis, and treatment of HIV-infected patients; high-risk behaviors; and an overview of the unique and complex psychosocial issues for the individual, the family, and the community.

Once all staff have been provided basic information about AIDS, the results of the needs assessment should be used to plan further education. All areas identified by staff as concerns or gaps in education should be addressed. As a general guideline, the clinical staff require information specific to their disciplines and the kind of care they are providing. A review of immunology and the immune system is helpful as an introduction to the many opportunistic infections that assault the person with AIDS. Subjects to be presented to clinical staff include: opportunistic infections; medications and treatments; symptom management; the drug and/or alcohol addicted patient; and a final session on ethical questions specific to hospice care of the HIV-infected patient, such as palliative versus curative care, maintaining hope, and accepting the hospice setting.

Special attention should be given to the issues unique to caring for AIDS patients at home. The patient needs to be protected from infections carried by other members of the household or visitors, including diseases such as colds, influenzas, or gastroenteritis. If the only available caregiver has an infection, he or she should wear a mask and adhere strictly to good handwashing procedures.

Because a varicella infection for a person with AIDS can have serious consequences, exposure of the patient to chicken pox is a special concern. If the patient has had chickenpox, it is less likely that reexposure to the virus will lead to complications. The risk of shingles, however, in the patient who has had chickenpox is significant enough that no one with chickenpox or no one recently exposed who has not previously had the disease should be allowed in the patient's room. Because more children than adults are susceptible to chickenpox, children should be screened carefully before visiting a patient with AIDS. A person with shingles should not care for the patient with AIDS until the shingles infection has subsided. If a patient with AIDS is exposed to chickenpox or shingles, the physician should be contacted immediately and prophylactic medication prescribed.

The re-emergence of tuberculosis (TB) as a public health concern is probably secondary to the HIV epidemic. HIV-related TB is notable in that it is one of the few associated infections that is communicable. It may manifest itself in unusual ways; for example, in the lymph nodes or in the lower portion of the lung. All persons with HIV infection and undiagnosed pulmonary disease should be suspected of having TB and appropriate precautions should be taken to prevent transmission until TB is ruled out or diagnosed and treated. Family caregivers with TB will need to be educated in preventing the transmission of TB, and others in the family will need to be tested for it. Hospice caregivers should participate in an ongoing TB screening program.

Other infection control issues include immunizations; pets; and gardening, food, and kitchen activities. Family teaching, always an important component of home care, becomes critically important when the elements of HIV infection and infection control are introduced.

Since the introduction of Medicare, home care has traditionally met the needs of the elderly for relatively low-technology care. The patient with AIDS, however, often requires "high-tech" treatment in the home. Examples are intravenous antibiotic therapy, parenteral nutrition, and blood transfusions. The course of AIDS is characterized by repeated episodes of crisis followed by periods of relative wellness. Care plans need to be adjusted frequently. This "roller coaster ride" can be extremely stressful to families, and they need skilled hospice staff to support them and to help them remain in control.

Once the staff have received their initial training in caring for patients with AIDS, it is important that they continue to receive current information about HIV infection and AIDS. The continuing education plan may include the use of periodicals, newsletters from local AIDS service organizations, speakers, films, seminars, and bulletin board presentations to keep staff informed.

Case Review

Regular, perhaps quarterly, review of a representative AIDS patient's use of hospice services can bring a personal and practical dimension to the education and updating of staff and can provide staff an opportunity to reopen problematic or unresolved issues. Case review is also helpful in the ongoing assessment of staff educational needs. The following format is suggested for conducting a case review. (See Figure 2.)

SUPERVISORY TRAINING

Crucial to the success of the program, as noted earlier, is the education provided to managers and supervisors. These staff set the tone for the response of the rest of the employees and volunteers

FIGURE 2. Format for Conducting Case Reviews

```
Attendance:      All clinical staff (home care and
                 inpatient); open to any other staff
                 who would like to attend

Time:            1-1/2 hours

Facilitator:     Person charged with responsibility for
                 HIV education plan

Format:          A. All team members participate in
                    presentation of patient information:
                       1. Diagnosis/presenting symptoms
                       2. Demographic information
                       3. Social history
                       4. Medical history
                       5. Course of hospice stay

                 B. All team members participate in
                    identification of problems
                       1. Resolved; solutions
                       2. Unresolved

                 C. All attendees participate in discussion

                 D. Representatives of as many services and
                    disciplines as possible present new
                    information about:
                       1. Treatments, medication
                       2. Nursing care (include inpatient if
                          indicated
                       3. Resources
                       4. Nutrition
                       5. Spiritual care
                       6. Bereavement care
                       7. Psychosocial issues
```

and, on a day-to-day basis, address the concerns of staff who care for AIDS patients. Managers and supervisors must also be prepared to respond to concerns raised by staff and to model acceptance of a worker who is HIV positive. Their training should precede and be separate from that of the rest of the staff. Their education plan should include an exploration of attitudes and feelings as well as the provision of information about disease symptoms and manifestations. When supervisors have been trained first, they can then assist in the training of other staff and can monitor compliance with universal precautions and infection control requirements.

Volunteers

Many hospice programs rely heavily on volunteers for patient care and for patient and family support. The type of education provided to volunteers should reflect their roles in the program. Volunteers who provide patient care should be included in any educational program about HIV infection and care of the person with AIDS. Although policy may require that an employee accept the assignment to care for an AIDS patient, this obligation may not apply to volunteers. Many volunteers, however, if appropriately educated and given the opportunity to address their preconceptions and concerns, are willing to be extremely supportive of the person with AIDS.

Responding to Families
of Traditional Hospice Patients

Family members of other patients may have concerns about the hospice program's acceptance of patients with HIV infection. A separate information/awareness program module may be prepared to be offered to these families. It may also be helpful for staff to talk with them on a one-to-one basis. It is important to provide factual information to allay fears about HIV transmission and to deal openly with negative feelings regarding homosexuality or intravenous drug use. Because interaction with someone who is open and nondefensive can accomplish a great deal in resolving this issue, an openly gay person, preferably a person with AIDS, may be asked to speak at an educational session for families of non-HIV-infected patients. Alternatively, a film on this topic may be shown, followed by a discussion period.

MONITORING COMPLIANCE

Quality Assurance

When policies are in place and training completed, the final step is to establish a process to ensure compliance. Research has shown that compliance with universal precautions and infection control may be less than optimal, even among highly trained professionals (Kearns, 1988). Quality assurance procedures, therefore, must include procedures for measuring compliance and taking corrective action if needed.

Staff who monitor compliance may consider examining the location of gowns and gloves to ensure that they are accessible, and to determine if personal protective equipment including nonallergenic gloves are available in the right sizes. The monitoring staff may also wish to look at infection control practices to determine if personal protective clothing is perhaps being overutilized. For example, gowning to bathe a patient or wearing gloves to serve food or sit with a patient wastes personal protective items and may cause distress to patients and their significant others. Other common deficiencies in infection control procedures include failing to change gloves or wash hands after patient contact and utilizing fluid-resistant gowns when it is unnecessary to do so. The best way to measure compliance with universal precautions is by direct observation. Repeated acts of noncompliance in certain areas may indicate a need for retraining or redesign of existing training programs and/or protocols.

Review of Staff Work Habits

Another aspect of monitoring compliance with infection control requirements is a review of staff work habits. The disposal of sharps, for instance, can be a great compliance problem. It is important to consider carefully both the location and type of sharps containers utilized to ensure maximal safety. Research shows that most needlestick injuries occur during recapping or disposal of sharps, even when an appropriate container is used (Jagger et al., 1988; White, 1990). This may be because the container is full and a needlestick occurs when disposing of the syringe, or because inconvenient placement of the container requires the nurse to handle the syringe and needle too long. The home care nurse needs to review whether supplies are readily available to household members and staff working in the home and needs to evaluate whether they are being properly used.

Housekeeping Practices

Other work practice controls that may require scrutiny and corrective action include housekeeping practices such as the handling of soiled laundry and cleanup and disposal of hazardous waste. All requirements pertaining to these areas are clearly spelled out in the proposed 1990 OSHA regulations.

Technological advances in equipment design are currently being looked to for improving protection of staff from occupational transmission of HIV and HBV (Jagger et al., 1988). The most significant recent development is the needleless syringe several variations of which are either already on or ready to enter the market. Staff who are responsible for purchasing such items should be encouraged to stay current with developments in this field and to explore all available options.

New policies and educational programs should be evaluated 3 to 6 months after implementation and thereafter annually. During the evaluation the following questions may be asked:

- Have CDC or OSHA recommendations changed?
- Are procedures consistent with policies?
- Does compliance indicate that training has been effective?
- Have issues or questions emerged that should be incorporated in policies?

CONCLUSION

Caring for patients with AIDS presents unique challenges to the hospice program, not only because of the complexity of the care, but also because of the issues surrounding the infectivity of the disease. Given the development of appropriate policies, however, and a comprehensive education and training program, caring for patients with AIDS can provide great satisfaction to the caregivers. Hospice care is an important element in the continuum of care for those with AIDS. A hospice program that is unprepared to respond when it learns that a staff member is infected with HIV faces an enormous challenge. Having policies in place and trained staff to deal with this issue before it arises is the best insurance that the organizational response will be, not only legally appropriate, but also demonstrative of the kindness and compassion that have been modeled so effectively for over a decade in the provision of hospice care to patients and families.

REFERENCES

Centers for Disease Control. (1987*a*). Recommendations for prevention of HIV transmission in health-care settings. *Morbidity and Mortality Weekly Report, 36* (Suppl. No. 2S).

Centers for Disease Control. (1987*b*). Update on hepatitis B prevention. *Morbidity and Mortality Weekly Report, 36*(23), 353-360, 366.

Centers for Disease Control. (1988). Update: universal precautions for prevention of transmission of human immunodeficiency virus, hepatitis B virus, and other bloodborne pathogens in health-care settings. *Morbidity and Mortality Weekly Report, 37*(24), 377-382, 387-388.

Jagger, J., Hunt, E., Brand-Elnaggar, J. & Pearson, R. (1988).

Rates of needle-stick injury caused by various devices in a university hospital. *New England Journal of Medicine, 319*(5), 284-287.

Kearns, K. P. (1988). Universal precautions: Employee resistance and strategies for planned organizational change. *Hospital and Health Services Administration, 33*(4), 521-530.

Marcus, R. & The CDC Cooperative Needlestick Surveillance Group. (1988). Surveillance of health care workers exposed to blood from patients infected with the human immunodeficiency virus. *New England Journal of Medicine, 319*(17), 1118-1123.

Occupational Safety and Health Administration. (1989). Occupational exposure to bloodborne pathogens. *Federal Register, 54*(102), 23134-23139.

Occupational Safety and Health Administration, Office of Health Compliance Assistance. (February 27, 1990). *Enforcement procedures for occupational exposure to hepatitis B virus (HBV) and human immunodeficiency virus (HIV).* (OSHA Instruction CPL 2-2.44B). Washington, DC: U. S. Government Printing Office.

White, K. (1990). "Why weren't you just more careful?" What does it take to avoid occupational exposure to HIV? *AIDS Patient Care*, *4*(3), 13-16.

BIBLIOGRAPHY
OF ADDITIONAL RESOURCE MATERIALS

Bay Area Symposium Business Leadership Task Force. (1986). *AIDS in the workplace*. San Francisco, CA: San Francisco AIDS Foundation.

Lewis, A. (1988). *Nursing care of the person with AIDS/ARC*. Rockville, MD: Aspen Publishers, Inc.

McGuirk, K. & Miles, T. (1987). Establishing a dedicated AIDS unit. *Journal of Nursing Administration*, *17*(6), 25-30.

Office of Personnel Management. (1988). *AIDS in the workplace policy*. (Bulletin NO. 792-42). Washington, DC: U.S. Government Printing Office.

Puckett, S. & Emory, A. (1988). *Managing AIDS in the workplace*. Reading, MA: Addison-Wesley Publishing Company.

AIDS
and the Hospice Community

"SLOW TRACK" = NEGATIVE PROGNOSTICATORS

"MEDIAN TRACK" = FOR IMMUNE SYSTEM FAILURE

"FAST TRACK" = POSITIVE PROGNOSTICATORS

"PROGNOSTICATORS" = P 24 ANTIGEN
BETA-2-MICROGLOBULIN
NEOPTERIN

STAGE I   STAGE II   STAGE III   STAGE IV   STAGE V   STAGE VI

PERCENT
OF
IMMUNE
SYSTEM
FUNCTION

20

Title: Parallel Issues for AIDS: Patients, Families and Others.

Authors: Ian Stulberg, Stephen Buckingham.

In: *Social Casework*, 69(6), June, 1988.

Key Issues: Identifies similar psychosocial issues faced by patients, families, significant others with treatment recommendations.

For Use By: Psychosocial Staff, Spiritual Care Staff, Volunteers, Care Coordinators/Managers.

Notes: Helpful both from conceptual as well as practical perspective for structuring adequate psychosocial care. Uses case examples and offers specific recommendations to help individuals and families.

Title: Women and AIDS: Countertransference Issues.

Author: Judy Macks.

In: *The Journal of Contemporary Social Work*, June, 1988.

Key Issues: Identifying countertransference reactions and recommendations to manage these reactions.

For Use By: Psychosocial Staff, Spiritual Care Staff, Nurse, Home Health Aides, Volunteers, Staff Support Facilitators.

Notes: Helpful in Assisting professional and volunteer caregivers manage their own responses, feelings, and needs triggered by the care of women with AIDS.

BOOKS

Title: *AIDS: The Drug and Alcohol Connector.*

Authors: Larry Siegel, MD, Milan Korcok.

Publisher: Hazelden Foundation, Center City, MN. 1989.

Key Issues: What professionals can do in treating AIDS and alcoholic and chemically dependent patients.

For Use By: Nurse Care Managers, Psychosocial Staff, Spiritual Care Staff, Care Coordinators/Managers.

Notes: From the Hazelden Group, which has done such pi-
                oneering and effective work in addiction. Addresses
                a much needed issue, especially Chapter 4 on the
                interface between drugs and AIDS, and Chapter 6
                on implementing care issues with chemically depen-
                dent patients.

Title: *The AIDS Caregiver Handbook.*
Author: Ted Eidson, Editor.
Publisher: St. Martin's Press, New York, NY, 1988.
Key Issues: Primary caregiver needs and issues.
For Use By: Primary Caregivers, Case Managers.
Notes: An excellent overview of all aspects of AIDS for
                caregivers, with especially helpful guidelines for
                home care, an explanation of grief and its impact,
                personal accounts from actual experiences of fam-
                ilies. Note: It is not hospice specific.

Title: *The AIDS Epidemic: Private Rights and the Public
                Interest.*
Author: Padraig O'Malley.
Publisher: Beacon Press, Boston, MA. 1989.
Key Issues: Public policy, status and implications, cost of care,
                reimbursement, confidentiality, list of resources.
For Use By: Administrators, Board Members.
Notes: Background to AIDS and public policy issues, with
                emphasis on reimbursements, confidentiality, costs
                of care; includes list of state by state resources.

Title: *The HIV Epidemic: New and Continuing Chal-
                lenges for the Public and Private Sector.*
Publisher: Council on Foundations Institute for Health Policy
                Studies, University of California, San Francisco,
                CA, 1989.
Key Issues: Public and private sector responses, financing and
                delivery of services, philanthropic role.
For Use By: Fund Raisers, Development Officers, Boards, Ad-
                ministrators.

Notes: Helpful in identifying the role of organized philanthropy in providing assistance and resources to help meet the health care crisis created by AIDS.

Title: *AIDS/HIV Infection: A Guide for Nursing Intervention*, 2nd Edition.
Author: Jacquelyn Flaskerud, Editor
Publisher: W.B. Saunders, Philadelphia, PA, 1989.
Key Issues: Nursing Care.
For Use By: Nurses, Nurse Managers/Supervisors.
Notes: Overall resource for nurses, with new section about home care and home care management.

Title: *Medical Management of AIDS*, 2nd Edition.
Author: Paul A. Volberding, MD.
Publisher: W.B. Saunders, Philadelphia, PA, 1990.
Key Issues: Up-to-date primary medical care.
For Use By: Medical Director, Medical Staff.
Notes: Practical resource for use by primary care physicians, medical directors, hospice physicians, and team coordinators/managers.

Title: *The Thirty-Six Hour Day*.
Authors: Nancy L. Mace, Peter V. Rabins, MD
Publisher: The Johns Hopkins University Press, Baltimore, MD, 1981.
Key Issues: Comprehensive overview of dementia, especially later stages.
For Use By: Professional Clinicians, Managers and Caregivers.
Notes: Though not AIDS specific, relevant for working with someone with dementia, especially the later stages.

JOURNALS

Title: AIDS and Families: Report of the AIDS Task Force Groves Conference on Marriage and the Family.

In: *Marriage and Family Review*, Vol. 13, The Haworth Press, Inc. 1989.
Key Issues: Impact of AIDS on traditional/nontraditional families.
For Use By: Nurse Managers, Psychosocial Staff, Spiritual Care Staff, Volunteers, Aides.
Notes: Written from a strong family systems framework, comprehensively treats issues of gay culture, substance abuse culture, differences in ethnic approaches to AIDS and bereavement. Touches all aspects.

Title: Healing A City.
Author: John Godges.
In: *Second Opinion*, The Park Ridge Center, Chicago, IL, Vol. 3, 1986.
Key Issues: Role of churches and voluntary organizations in San Francisco.
For Use By: Psychosocial Staff, Spiritual Care Staff.
Notes: From the creative and innovative Park Ridge Center, reviews critical role of churches in assisting with the creating of the so-called "San Francisco model" and the religious issues involved with gay men.

Title: The Spectrum of HIV Infection in Adults.
In: *Seminars in Oncology Nursing*, Vol. 5, No. 4, November, 1989.
Key Issues: Epidemiology, prevention, treatment strategies, nursing issues, psychosocial issues.
For Use By: Nurses.
Notes: Excellent comprehensive overview for nurses of a wide range of information, including current treatment strategies, lymphomas, care for Kaposi's Sarcoma, mental health issues, symptom management, and psychosocial and cultural issues.

MANUALS

Title: *AIDS: A Self-Care Manual.*
Publisher: IBS Press, Santa Monica, CA, 1987.
Contact: 213-450-6485
Key Issues: Terminal care, spiritual care, psychosocial issues.
For Use By: Patients, Family Members, Nurse and Psychosocial Case Managers, Spiritual Care Providers.
Notes: Developed as a self-help tool for patients and their primary caregivers, this manual is also helpful for all clinicians and volunteers. Includes chapters by persons who have been caregivers of AIDS patients. Also includes helpful information on legal concerns, support options, spiritual issues, terminal care issues.

Title: *AIDS: Home Care and Hospice Manual*, 2nd Edition.
Publisher: Visiting Nurses Association of San Francisco, CA. San Francisco, 1990.
Contact: 415-861-8705
Key Issues: Thorough revision of most complete and comprehensive guide to home care and hospice services for persons with AIDS.
For Use By: Interdisciplinary Managers and Clinicians.
Notes: Especially helpful for programs with limited AIDS experience as well as an update on current practice for more experienced teams. Covers infection control, assessment, nursing intervention, psychosocial care, care issues for caregivers, substance abuse, and bereavement.

Title: *A North American Conference on Care of Terminally Ill Persons with AIDS.*
Publisher: National Hospice Organization, Arlington, VA, 1987.
Contact: 703-243-5900
Key Issues: Comprehensive range of issues including psychosocial, spiritual, nursing, bereavement, support for

caregivers.

For Use By: Nurses, Psychosocial Staff, Spiritual Care Staff, Bereavement Staff, Aides, Volunteers.

Notes: Includes papers from wide range of experts presented at conference sponsored by the National Hospice Organization. Excellent source of background materials, general education, and specific care guidelines and issues across all disciplines and services. Valuable in that it is hospice specific.

Title: *Developing AIDS Residential Settings.*

Publisher: Visiting Nurses Association of San Francisco, CA, San Francisco, CA, 1988.

Contact: 415-861-8705.

Key Issues: Step-by-step planning guidelines for creating an AIDS residence. Presents resources, alternatives, and planning material.

For Use By: Administrators, Board Members, Key Planners.

Notes: Utilizes the experience of Coming Home Hospice of San Francisco. Well-organized and comprehensive A to Z manual of how to do it and what the alternatives are.

Title: *Guidelines for Caring for Persons with AIDS.*

Publisher: National Hospice Organization, Arlington, VA, 1987.

Contact: 703-243-5900

Key Issues: Hospice-Specific Comprehensive Guidelines.

For Use By: Nurses, Psychosocial Staff, Spiritual Care Staff, Aides, Volunteers.

Notes: Specifically written by hospice professionals for hospice professionals and volunteers, provides much helpful and detailed specific information of value to all team members. Includes guidelines for psychosocial and nursing interventions, bereavement support, staff support.

Title: *Working with AIDS: A Resource Guide for Mental Health Workers.*

Publisher: University of California at San Francisco, CA, June, 1987.
Contact: 415-476-6430
Key Issues: Training, interventions, resources for mental health professionals working with AIDS related issues.
For Use By: Psychosocial Staff, Spiritual Care Providers.
Notes: Very helpful material for psychosocial and spiritual care providers and their managers, with much information transferable to both nurse case managers and volunteers. Not hospice specific.

NEWSLETTER

Title: *AIDS Health Project*.
Publisher: University of California at San Francisco, CA, Monthly.
Contact: 415-476-6430
Key Issues: A guide to AIDS research, care, counseling.
For Use By: Care Team Managers and Professionals.
Notes: Provides timely information on new treatment strategies, new experimental initiatives, as well as resources for wide-ranging care issues.

AUDIOTAPES

Title: *Counseling the PWA Couple*.
90 Minutes
Producer: National Lesbian and Gay Health Foundation. Washington, DC, 1988.
Contact: National Audiovisual Transcript, 800-373-2952, No. XI-24.
Key Issues: Interventions for couples facing grieving, guilt, financial change, sexuality.
For Use By: Psychosocial Staff, Volunteers, Spiritual Care Staff.
Notes: Gays speaking about their own experiences. Very helpful for hospices whose AIDS case load includes

gay couples. Uses sexually explicit language, and involves issues of grief, self-blame, financial stresses, social upheaval, sexuality.

Title:	*Grieving Our Losses: AIDS and Bereavement.* 90 Minutes
Producer:	National Lesbian and Gay Health Foundation, Washington, DC, 1989.
Contact:	Learn to Listen Tape Library, San Diego, CA 800-537-8273.
Key Issues:	Discussion by persons doing grief work, interventions. Discusses the advisability of using stage-model.
For Use By:	Psychosocial Staff, Spiritual Care Provider, Bereavement, Staff Volunteers.
Notes:	Presents ways of supporting grief work of persons within the context of AIDS. (Staff of the Whitman Walker Clinic in Washington, DC). Special attention is paid to practitioners who may work out a rigid stage model of grief that may not be appropriate. Includes sexually explicit language.

Title:	*HIV Counseling: Issues for the Psychotherapist.* 90 Minutes
Producer:	National Lesbian and Gay Health Foundation, Washington, DC, 1989.
Contact:	Listen to Learn Tape Library, San Diego, CA, 619-569-1333.
Key Issues:	Countertransference, empowerment, intervention, differences of HIV population.
For Use By:	Psychosocial Staff, Spiritual Care Provider, Volunteers.
Notes:	Helpful clinical model using stages of HIV disease process, risk factors, and ecology map of HIV client/patient. Special attention is paid to countertransference, issues of fear, denial, and over-identification, and quality of life issues.

Title: *Intimacy and AIDS: Issues of Love, Loss and Lone-
                liness for Gay Men.*
                90 Minutes
Producer: National Lesbian and Gay Health Foundation,
                Washington, DC, 1988.
Contact: National Audiovisual Transcript, 800-373-2952,
                Order No. VIII-15.
Key Issues: Interventions for dealing with impact of AIDS upon
                intimate relationships and behaviors.
For Use By: Psychosocial Staff, Spiritual Care Provider, Volun-
                teers, Care Managers/Coordinators.
Notes: Very helpful in sensitizing clinical staff. Addresses
                impact of AIDS stigma on relationships, with spe-
                cial detailed attention to fear of isolation and rejec-
                tion. Examines how patients perceive, process and
                integrate these adjustments. Sexually explicit lan-
                guage.

Title: *Perspectives on Suicide and AIDS/HIV.*
                90 Minutes
Producer: National Lesbian and Gay Health Foundation,
                Washington, DC, 1989.
Contact: Listen to Learn Tape Library, San Diego, CA, 619-
                569-1333.
Key Issues: Risk factors, stages of suicidal contemplation, inter-
                ventions.
For Use By: Nurses, Psychosocial Staff, Spiritual Care Staff,
                Volunteers, Care Managers/Coordinators.
Notes: Excellent presentation on experience of suicide
                within the AIDs trajectory. Includes very detailed
                and specific assessment and intervention ap-
                proaches. Presents the Shanti Project model.

Title: *Significant Others Support Groups.*
                90 Minutes
Producer: National Lesbian and Gay Health Foundation,
                Washington, DC, 1988.

Contact: National Audiovisual Transcript, Order No. III 6, 800-373-2952
Key Issues: Stigma, guilt, quality of life, anger, secretiveness, decision-making, loss, hope, primarily for gay caregivers.
For Use By: Psychosocial Staff, Spiritual Care Provider, Volunteers, Care Managers.
Notes: Information about issues and needs of caregivers of AIDS patients, especially gay partners; includes emotional issues, legal issues, and ethical issues; sexually explicit language.

VIDEOTAPES

Title: AIDS Home Care and Hospice Video.
                  35 Minutes
Producer: Visiting Nurses and Hospice of San Francisco, CA, 1989.
Contact: 415-998-5332.
Key Issues: Training Film for Interdisciplinary Team, especially nurses; home management stressed; includes patient/caregiver interventions.
For Use By: Interdisciplinary Team Volunteers, Care Managers/ Coordinators.
Notes: Utilizes the experience of the Visiting Nurses Hospice of San Francisco. Especially helpful in demonstrating a continuum of disability for persons with AIDS; specific information related to physical interventions necessary for AIDS hospice home care; an overview of psychosocial considerations; shows photographs of actual patient/caregiver interactions.

Title: *AIDS: A Mirror of Loneliness.*
                  39 Minutes
Producer: New York University, AIDS Education and Training Center, 1989.
Contact: 212-998-5332.
Key Issues: English and Spanish (Puerto Rican). Patients' per-

spectives; emphasizes value of communication.

For Use By:	Interdisciplinary Team, Volunteers, Care Managers/Coordinators.
Notes:	Helpful for agencies with Puerto Ricans on the AIDS caseload. Addresses cultural, ethical, attitudinal barriers to communications and relationships.

Title:	*Circle of Warriors, Part 1.* 26 Minutes
Producer:	Seattle Indian Health Board, 1989.
Contact:	206-324-9360.
Key Issues:	Native Americans with AIDS; cultural issues.
For Use By:	Interdisciplinary Team, especially Psychosocial Staff, Care Managers/Coordinators.
Notes:	Very helpful presentation of issues of Native American pride and self-concept, and the impact of this upon Native Americans with AIDS; for agencies whose caseloads involve them or ought to involve them in the care of Native Americans.

Title:	*Common Threads: Stories from the Quilt.* 75 Minutes
Producer:	Telling Pictures, Inc., Namely Project, San Francisco, CA, 1989.
Contact:	415-863-5511
Key Issues:	Stories recounted by families and loved ones; homophobia, public policy.
For Use By:	Broad use: Board, Clinical Staff, Volunteers, Care Managers/Coordinators.
Notes:	Very moving. Emphasizes the human dimensions of AIDS by focusing on family members and loved ones as they tell their stories of individuals memorialized on the Quilt. Places the personal experience within the context of society's response.

Title:	*Finding Our Way Together: People with AIDS and Their Caregivers.* 28 Minutes
Producer:	American Red Cross, Seattle, WA, 1989.

Contact: 206-323-2345
Key Issues: Thirty anecdotes about how HIV/AIDS affects peo-
                ple's lives and relationships; Church roles.
For Use By: Broad use: Board, Clinical Staff, Volunteers, Care
                Managers/Coordinators.
Notes: Excellent production of a series of vignettes as 30
                people; caregivers, church members, professionals,
                patients, and a foster mother talk about their experi-
                ence with AIDS. Emphasizes living with the disease
                rather than dying from it. Sexually explicit lan-
                guage.

Title: *Pediatric AIDS: A Time of Crisis*.
                23 Minutes
Producer: Association for the Care of Children's Health,
                Washington, DC, 1989.
Contact: 301-654-6549
Key Issues: Descriptions of children's families; Hispanics,
                Afro-Americans.
For Use By: Psychosocial Staff, Spiritual Care Staff, Volun-
                teers, Care Managers/Coordinators.
Notes: Especially helpful as a cross-cultural, cross-racial
                presentation of both biological families' and foster
                families' experiences with pediatric AIDS, includ-
                ing when parents also are infected. Describes the
                comprehensive, flexible program Albert Einstein
                Hospital, Bronx, New York has developed.

Title: *Too Little, Too Late*.
                48 Minutes
Producer: Fanlight Productions, Boston, MA, 1987.
Contact: 617-524-0980
Key Issues: Candid interviews; distressing symptoms; supports;
                stress.
For Use By: Interdisciplinary Team, Volunteers, Board.
Notes: Interviews with persons with AIDS and family
                members. Covers death and dying issues, stress, re-
                jection, isolation, coping with dementia, blindness,

and premature aging. Emphasizes need for openness, honesty and support. Gay focus for patients.

Title: *Mildred Pearson: When You Love a Person.*
            10 Minutes
Producer: Video Data Bank, New York, NY, 1989.
Contact: 212-233-3441
Key Issues: Story of Afro-American Family Caring for Son; Explicit language, stress, terminal care.
For Use By: Board, Staff, Volunteers.
Notes: A mother's story of the life and death of her son from AIDS, emphasizing the emotional impact upon her. Helps in creating cultural understanding and sensitivity.

BOOK REVIEW

Title: *AIDS/HIV Infection: A Reference Guide for Nursing Professionals*
Author: Jacquelyn Haak Flaskerud, RN, PhD, FAAP
Publisher: W.B. Saunders Company, Philadelphia, PA, 1989.
Reviewer: Virginia Shubert, RN, MN
Summary: This is a basic reference guide for nurses involved in the primary, secondary, and tertiary prevention and treatment of HIV infection.
Major Points: The overview of AIDS/HIV history; sociodemographic distribution (world-wide to 2/88) and risk factors; description of normal immune system function and the impact of HIV infection; tables of common opportunistic infections; drug therapies and drug side effects; nursing care plans for common AIDS/ARC symptoms; discussion of psycho-social, ethical and legal aspects of AIDS care; community issues in prevention and treatment of HIV infection and comprehensive listing of AIDS hotlines and care resources (state, national and international); listing of state and territorial departments of health and contacts for a wide range of educational materi-

als, directories and newsletters; appendices reporting the 1988 CDC Surveillance case definition for prevention of HIV transmission in health care settings are extremely informative. The tones of all chapter authors are knowledgeable and compassionate: terms offensive to the majority of persons with AIDS, such as "AIDS victims" are NEVER used. The reality of impaired nursing care based on fear and prejudices held by many professionals is acknowledged and HEALTHY coping and self-care practices are explicitly encouraged.

Weaknesses: This book is not, nor does it claim to be, a clinical practice manual. Most information on opportunistic infections and standard treatments is available elsewhere. Complex symptom management and treatment decisions are not addressed. Hospice care of persons with AIDS is not a primary focus of this book and the complex issues of cost/benefit analysis for care of the terminally ill are not addressed in any depth.

For Use By: This book is a good reference for any program developing AIDS care policies. It serves as a useful tool in reviewing existing general policies with an eye to updating them. Finally, its resource access guide is comprehensive.

Index